DEVELOPING INNOVATIVE COMMUNITY-BASED LONG-TERM CARE SYSTEMS AND SERVICES

NOVEMBER 2025

ASIAN DEVELOPMENT BANK

6 ADB Avenue, Mandaluyong City, 1550 Metro Manila, Philippines
Tel +63 2 8632 4444; Fax +63 2 8636 2444
www.adb.org

ISBN 978-92-9277-503-2 (print); 978-92-9277-504-9 (PDF); 978-92-9277-505-6 (ebook)
Publication Stock No. TCS250454-2
DOI: http://dx.doi.org/10.22617/TCS250454-2

Notes:
In this publication, "MNT" refers to Mongolian togrog and "$" refers to United States dollars.
ADB recognizes "China" as the People's Republic of China.

On the cover: Mbah Djariyah does needlework in her home in Yogyakarta, Indonesia. Home-based and community-based care programs address older people's needs for assistance with everyday activities. (photo by Anita Reza Zein/ADB).

Printed on recycled paper

Contents

Tables, Figures, and Boxes iv

Foreword v

Acknowledgments vii

Abbreviations viii

Introduction 1

Long-Term Care Trends and Systems in Indonesia, Mongolia, and Viet Nam 4

- Increasing Prevalence of Frailty and Noncommunicable Diseases in an Aging Population 4
- Functional Impairment and Loss of Independence in Daily Living 5
- Fragile and Underdeveloped Long-Term Care Systems 5
- Policy Improvements 6

Rationale for Investing in Community-Based Long-Term Care 7

Regional Pilot to Develop Community-Based Long-Term Care Systems and Services 9

Models of Care 11

- Three Contexts, Three Models of Care 11

Community-Based Long-Term Care Workforce 27

- Management, Health, and Social Care Workforce 27
- Indispensable Role of Family Caregivers 28
- Volunteers Are a Valuable Asset 29
- Capacity Building 30

Innovation and Technology in Long-Term Care in the Pilot 33

- Digital Care and Case Management 33
- Data Utilization 33

Health and Social Care Integration 34

- Connecting to the Larger Ecosystem 34

Key Successes 38

Key Lessons Learned 40

Strategic Recommendations 43

Tables, Figures, and Boxes

TABLES

1 Aging Population and Impairment Rates in Indonesia, Mongolia, and Viet Nam 5
2 Community-Based Long-Term Care Model 10
3 Service-Matching Recommendations 15
4 Prevalence of Care Foci Among Older Adults Classified as Level 3, with Viet Nam as an Example 17
5 Training Programs Developed 31

FIGURES

1 Case Management Flow 14
2 Indonesia's Community Care Hub Model 19
3 Active Aging Hub Model 22
4 Stakeholder Mapping and Structure of Viet Nam's Care Model 24
5 How Integrated Care Is Achieved Through Case Management 35
6 Combining the ICOPE Approach with Pilot Care Model 37

BOXES

1 What Is Community-Based Long-Term Care? 2
2 World Health Organization ICOPE Approach 36

Foreword

Over half of the global population aged 60 years and above reside in Asia and the Pacific, and the number is projected to rise to approximately 1.3 billion by 2050. Population aging has major economic and social implications, including raising concerns about who will provide care for growing numbers of older people with more long-term and complex care needs. Currently, most care provision to older people is supplied informally by family members, who rarely receive any support or training. As population demographics change, there is a need to develop systems and services to help alleviate the widening gap between demand and supply, and provide quality services.

Population aging has major economic and social implications, including raising concerns about who will provide care for growing numbers of older people with more long-term and complex care needs.

Starting in 2016, the Asian Development Bank (ADB) worked with the governments of Indonesia, Mongolia, Sri Lanka, Thailand, Tonga, and Viet Nam to understand the current situation in long-term care (LTC), identify good practices and gaps, and help map out the road ahead to meet the challenge of growing demand for LTC. All studied countries favored supporting older people to stay in their homes and communities—known as aging in place—rather than to go into residential care.

In these countries, nongovernment, civil society, and faith-based organizations are providing care for older people in their homes and in the community, but demand outstrips supply. Residential care is not widely available and is often expensive and beyond the means of most of the population. Developing effective, low-cost care models that can be replicated or scaled up, and building evidence based on the impact of investments, are important steps to developing LTC systems in the region. These systems have wide-ranging influence because LTC is a core component of both the health and social service sectors. Its development also has significant implications for job creation, and the demand for education and training. It can help promote gender equity by recognizing the contribution of female caregivers and the economic vulnerabilities of older women.

In December 2019, ADB approved the regional knowledge and support technical assistance project, Developing Innovative Community-Based Long-Term Care Systems and Services, to design and develop innovative, affordable, and sustainable community-based LTC service models in rural and urban areas that respond to the care needs of older people and build on the contexts and strengths of existing social and health care services in Indonesia, Mongolia, and Viet Nam. The project recognized four priorities: developing integrated health and social care services, creating case management systems to facilitate integration, promoting healthy and active aging, and enhancing human resource development of both formal and informal carers.

Highlighting the experiences of the community-based LTC pilot projects in the three selected countries, this publication intends to offer pathways for other countries to embark on developing their respective LTC systems and services. We believe that the country challenges, lessons learned, and recommendations summarized in the report can offer invaluable insights to policymakers and various stakeholders across the region. ADB stands ready to collaborate with its developing member countries as they endeavor to provide integrated care and services to their growing population of older people.

Eduardo Banzon
Director, Human and Social Development Sector Office
Sectors Department 3, Asian Development Bank

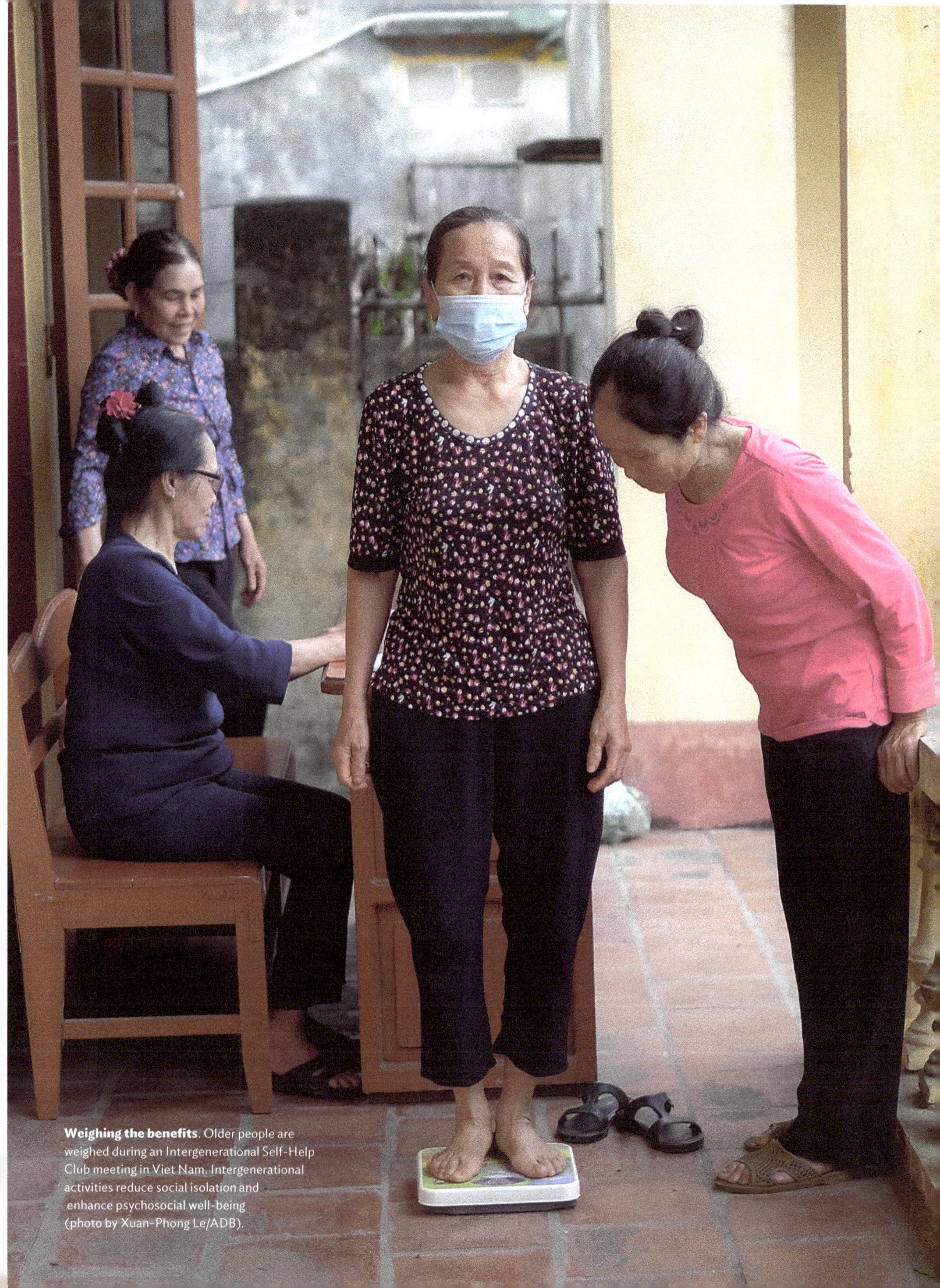

Weighing the benefits. Older people are weighed during an Intergenerational Self-Help Club meeting in Viet Nam. Intergenerational activities reduce social isolation and enhance psychosocial well-being (photo by Xuan-Phong Le/ADB).

Acknowledgments

This report summarizes the findings and lessons learned from the implementation of the regional technical assistance (TA) project, Developing Innovative Community-Based Long-Term Care Systems and Services. The initiative was funded by the High-Level Technology Fund, the Japan Fund for Prosperous and Resilient Asia and the Pacific, the Japan Special Fund, and the Asian Development Bank (ADB) Technical Assistance Special Fund. ADB is grateful to the governments of Indonesia, Mongolia, and Viet Nam for their cooperation—particularly our counterpart teams from the Ministry of National Development Planning/National Development Planning Agency (Bappenas) of Indonesia; the Ministry of Family, Labour and Social Protection of Mongolia; and the Ministry of Health of Viet Nam—for their commitment to advancing this initiative.

The following ADB staff and consultants supported the implementation of the TA and provided inputs into the preparation of this report: Rachanichol Arunoprayote, Putu Suka Aryana, Nguyen Ngoc Bich, Enkhtsetseg Byambaa, Putu Darma, Lydia Domingo, Altantuya Jigjidsuren, Itgel Longid, Imelda Marquez, Emiko Masaki, Sri Mulyani, Vinh Ngo, Astrid Nikijuluw, Nyamgerel Oyunbat, Heru Subekti, Deeny Uli Rosa Simanjuntak, Arlene Tadle, Sakiko Tanaka, Bui Dai Thu, Tran Bich Thuy, Nong Thi Thu Trang, and Sani Utami. Special thanks to Najibullah Habib, principal health specialist, Human and Social Development Sector Office, Sectors Department 3 (SD3-HSD) for serving as the peer reviewer for this report. The TA also benefited from the overall guidance of Wendy Walker, former director, and Meredith Wyse, former senior social development specialist (aging and care), SD3-HSD. Finalization and completion of this report and the TA's other deliverables have been led by Emiko Masaki, principal health specialist, SD3-HSD.

Writers: Peter Chan, Ng Wai Chong, Jane Parry, Meredith Wyse
Copy editor: Maria Theresa Mercado
Layout and design: Solveig Bang, Rocilyn Laccay
Proofreader: Lawrence Casiraya

Abbreviations

AAH	active aging hub
ADB	Asian Development Bank
ADL	activities of daily living
CCH	community care hub
DMC	developing member country
IADL	instrumental activities of daily living
ICOPE	Integrated Care for Older People
ISHC	Intergenerational Self-Help Club
LTC	long-term care
NCD	noncommunicable disease
NGO	nongovernment organization
SILANI	Elderly Information System
WHO	World Health Organization

Introduction

International experience and evidence show that the best way to manage demand for care and support services for older adults is through community-based long-term care and an integrated approach bringing together health, social, and other sectors.

Asia and the Pacific is a fast-aging region. The number of people aged 60 and above is projected to almost double, from 670 million people in 2022 to 1.3 billion people by 2050.[1] They will also account for a greater proportion of the region's total population: one in every four people, up from one in seven in 2022. Women are disproportionately represented among older adults, accounting for 54% of the population aged 60 and above, a share that increases with age due to women's longer life expectancy.

The overall decrease in poverty in developing Asian economies includes a reduction in poverty among older adults, but they may not benefit as much as younger family members because family resources are not distributed equally. Also, they grapple with noncommunicable diseases (NCDs) and heightened loneliness and social isolation. These challenges are exacerbated by suboptimal access to essential services. International experience and evidence show that the best way to manage demand for care and support services for older adults is through community-based long-term care (LTC) and an integrated approach bringing together health, social, and other sectors (Box 1).

The Asian Development Bank (ADB) is supporting its developing member countries (DMCs) to prepare for this demographic change in a variety of ways, including financial and technical support to develop new models of community-based LTC for older adults. The aim is to identify models that are affordable, sustainable, and appropriate, and best meet the needs of older adults and their families in the unique context of each country in the region. The lessons generated from ADB projects are being used to inform national policies and programs.

This report examines the results of a regional technical assistance project that brought innovative, community-based LTC models to three countries with different contexts: Indonesia, Mongolia and Viet Nam.[2] The models were rooted in a global body of evidence that supports community-based LTC and an integrated approach. These frame aging beyond the biomedical model, to incorporate social, economic, and physical well-being. They promote active aging in place and respect the caregiving traditions of each country, while adapting to changing social structures. Through pilot projects in each of the three countries, important lessons were learned that can inform not only each country's own social policy, but also those of other countries in Asia and the Pacific, and beyond.

This report outlines LTC trends and challenges in Indonesia, Mongolia, and Viet Nam, with detailed descriptions of the pilot models. There are dedicated sections on the role of both human resources and technology in the provision of community-based LTC. Finally, there is a discussion of each pilot project's key successes, lessons learned, and strategic recommendations for replication and scale-up.

---

1 United Nations Economic and Social Commission for Asia and the Pacific (UNESCAP). 2022. *Asia-Pacific Report on Population Ageing 2022: Trends, policies and good practices regarding older persons and population ageing.*

2 ADB. 2019. Technical Assistance for Developing Innovative Community-Based Long-Term Care Systems and Services (TA 9228-REG).

Box 1: What Is Community-Based Long-Term Care?

The World Health Organization (WHO) defines long-term care (LTC) as "the activities undertaken by others to ensure that people with or at risk of a significant ongoing loss of intrinsic capacity can maintain a level of functional ability consistent with their basic rights, fundamental freedoms and human dignity."[a] When people have functional ability, they can meet their basic needs; learn, grow, and make decisions; be mobile; build and maintain relationships; and contribute to society.[b]

Implicit in the WHO definition of LTC is the promotion of a holistic, person-centered approach and early intervention for older people at risk of unmet needs for complex care. LTC encompasses both health and social care and support, aiming to enhance quality of life and maintain independence as much as possible.

LTC primarily serves older adults, but it also includes younger individuals with disabilities or chronic conditions. It can be provided in various environments, including institutions such as nursing homes and assisted living facilities. WHO defines community-based LTC as a form of formal, non-residential LTC that is provided and organized at the community level.

[a] WHO. 2015. *World Report on Ageing and Health*.
[b] WHO. 2019. *Decade of Healthy Ageing 2020–2030*.
Source: Compiled by author.

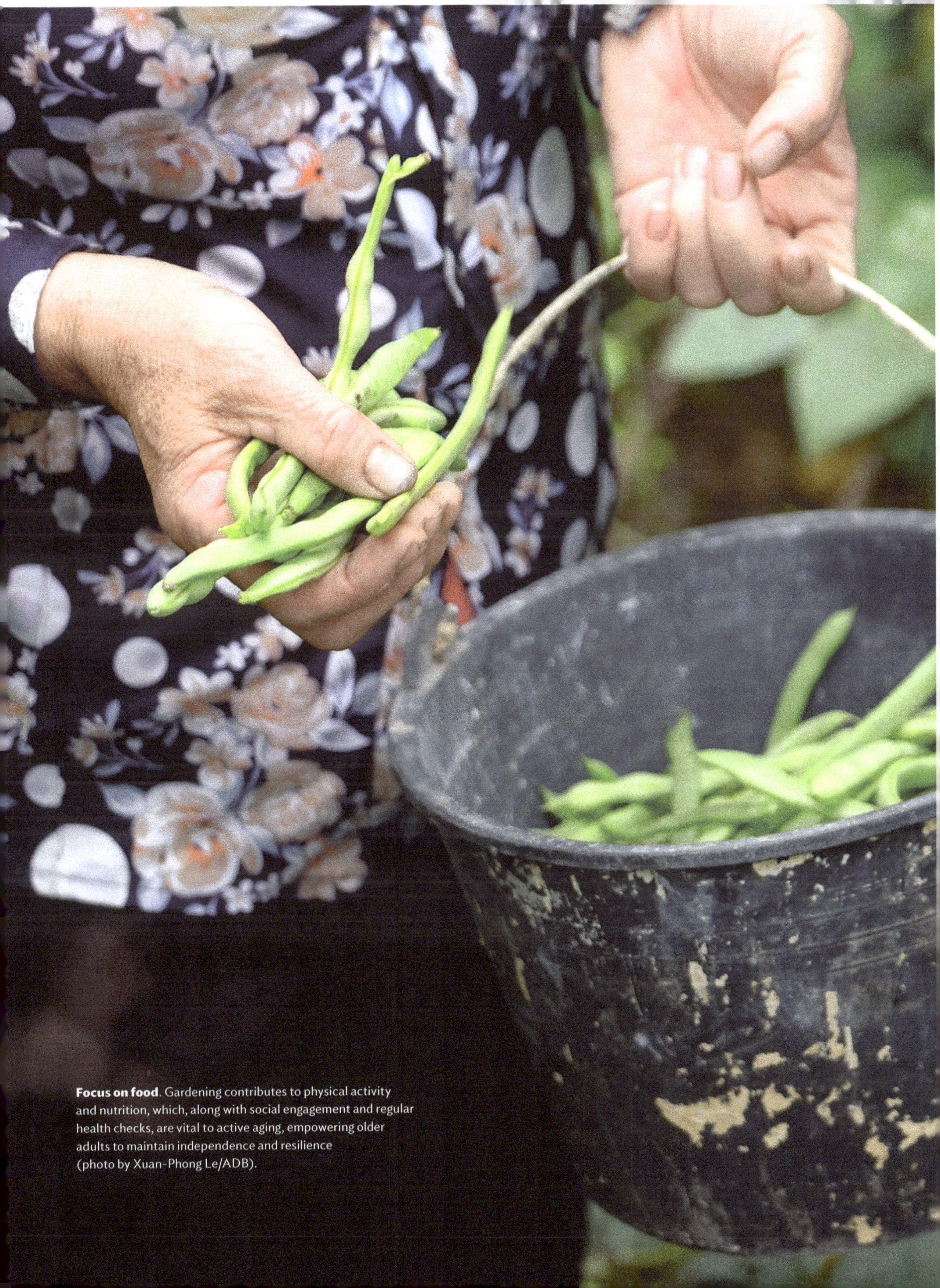

Focus on food. Gardening contributes to physical activity and nutrition, which, along with social engagement and regular health checks, are vital to active aging, empowering older adults to maintain independence and resilience (photo by Xuan-Phong Le/ADB).

Long-Term Care Trends and Systems in Indonesia, Mongolia, and Viet Nam

The demographic landscape of Indonesia, Mongolia, and Viet Nam is marked by a rapid increase in their aging populations at varying rates. This shift, coupled with the rise of NCDs and the increasing prevalence of frailty, creates a complex set of challenges to their health and social care systems, ultimately leading to increased disability and the need for LTC.

Most developing countries face a double disease burden, confronting both infectious diseases and the growing wave of noncommunicable diseases that contribute toward the development of disabilities, including cognitive impairment and dementia.

Indonesia has a relatively young older population but is also on an upward trajectory, with the population aged 60 and above projected to rise from 10% in 2019 to 21% by 2050.[3] Mongolia's population will remain relatively young overall, but the proportion aged 60 and above is expected to more than double in 30 years, from 7.2% in 2020 to 17.3% in 2050 (in Mongolia, older adults are defined as women aged 55 and above, and men aged 60 and above).[4] Viet Nam is experiencing the most rapid aging process. In 2019, 11.9% of the population were aged 60 and above, but by 2050 the proportion is forecast to rise to 25%.[5]

Increasing Prevalence of Frailty and Noncommunicable Diseases in an Aging Population

As human cells age, they accumulate damage and become less able to perform their usual functions. Thus, as people age, physiological deficiencies accumulate resulting in a declining health and increasing susceptibility to adverse health outcomes, including the development of NCDs. This state of increased risk of adverse health outcomes due to an accumulation of deficits is one way of understanding frailty.[6]

Thus, an aging population and frailty in advanced age, combined with lifestyle changes and urbanization, are driving a surge in NCDs across Indonesia, Mongolia, and Viet Nam.[7] Globally, NCDs account for 75% of deaths, and 73% of all NCD deaths are in developing countries.[8] Most developing countries face a double disease burden, confronting both infectious diseases and the growing wave of NCDs that contribute toward the development of disabilities, including cognitive impairment and dementia.

---

3 ADB. 2022. *The Road to Better Long-Term Care in Asia and the Pacific.*

4 Government of Mongolia, National Statistical Office. 2020. *Population Projection Based on Housing and Population Census.*

5 United Nations Population Fund. Viet Nam.

6 K. Rockwood and A. Mitnitski. 2011. Frailty defined by deficit accumulation and geriatric medicine defined by frailty. *Clinics in Geriatric Medicine.* 27(1). pp. 7–26.

7 ADB. 2023. *Local Mapping and Needs Assessment Report, Viet Nam.* April.

8 World Health Organization (WHO). 2024. Noncommunicable diseases.

Functional Impairment and Loss of Independence in Daily Living

NCDs are the leading causes of disability in performing the activities of daily living (ADLs), such as bathing, dressing, eating, and mobility, as well as the instrumental activities of daily living (IADLs) like managing finances or medication. Many DMCs struggle with NCD prevention, diagnosis, and management, as well as providing access to adequate LTC. In Indonesia, Mongolia, and Viet Nam, 10%–25% of older adults experience ADL or IADL impairment, often linked to untreated NCDs and sensory losses, and exacerbated by frailty (Table 1).

Socioeconomic factors, such as gender inequality, limited education, and poverty, further compound these challenges.

Table 1. Aging Population and Impairment Rates in Indonesia, Mongolia, and Viet Nam

Country	Population ≥60 (2024 Estimate)	Proportion of Total Population	Frailty Prevalence (≥60)	NCD Prevalence (≥60)	ADL Impairment Rate (≥60)
Indonesia	~31.8 million	~11.5%	~10%–15% (estimated)	60%–70%	30% (10% severely impaired)
Mongolia	~0.32 million	~9.2%	10%–15%	~60% (estimated)	25% (7% severely impaired)
Viet Nam	~13.5 million	~13.7%	~12%–20% (estimated)	~60% (estimated)	~45% (22% - 2+ ADL impairment)

ADL = activities of daily living, NCD = noncommunicable disease.

Data sources: The Lancet. Global Burden of Disease; UN Department of Economic and Social Affairs. Data on Older Persons; World Health Organization (WHO). 2024. World Health Statistics. Monitoring health for the SDGs, Sustainable Development Goals; WHO. 2025. Aging Data Portal: Maternal, Newborn, Child and Adolescent Health and Ageing. 3 May; Asian Development Bank (ADB). 2021. *Diagnostic Study on Long-Term Care in Indonesia*; R. W. Basrowi et al. 2021. The Road to Healthy Ageing: What Has Indonesia Achieved So Far? *Nutrients*. 13(10). p. 3441; ADB. 2020. *Country Diagnostic Study on Long-Term Care in Mongolia*; ADB. 2017. Country Diagnostic Study on Long-Term Care in Viet Nam (1st draft). November.

Source: Compiled by authors.

Fragile and Underdeveloped Long-Term Care Systems

Across Indonesia, Mongolia, and Viet Nam, informal, family-based care and the use of volunteers remain the cornerstones of support for older adults. This tradition, deeply rooted in cultural values, provides a cost-effective lifeline and reinforces family and community solidarity, but fails to address fundamental societal shifts. Shrinking family size, urban migration, and the growing complexity of care needs are challenging the capacity of families and volunteers to shoulder this burden alone. Family caregivers provide invaluable emotional and practical support, but face psychological stress, and lack respite care, training, and community and government support (footnote 8).

The LTC systems that do exist are generally reactive, responding to requests for service. They lack resources and are ill-equipped to identify at-risk older adults and address their complex care needs. The roles of different types of care providers from the health and social welfare sectors frequently overlap, and integration is limited at best. Many older adults and their caregivers struggle to manage mobility issues and chronic conditions like dementia, and there is a critical need for psychosocial support services.

Models for LTC have emerged in Indonesia, Mongolia, and Viet Nam, but they all have room for improvement. Indonesia's robust cadre network, while providing community health and social functions serving millions, requires more expertise and infrastructure to address complex care needs. Only certain types of cadres are specifically tasked with care support for older adults and their families, leaving families and untrained caregivers overburdened. However, future efforts can build on the strong experience of the cadre network. Viet Nam's Intergenerational Self-Help Clubs (ISHCs) blend community engagement with care. Scaling these clubs and integrating them with professional support could amplify their impact. In Mongolia, LTC systems, rooted in medical and rehabilitative services, have the potential to evolve into more holistic models by incorporating continuous care and addressing social and emotional well-being.

By building on these strengths—integrating multidisciplinary professionals, improving resource allocation, and fostering collaboration across the services introduced by the pilot projects—these countries can create scalable, person-centered LTC systems. Such systems would not only meet the rising demand for care but also ensure older adults thrive with dignity and support.

Policy Improvements

Recognizing the urgency of the situation, Indonesia, Mongolia, and Viet Nam have all made some strides in policy development.

- **Indonesia**: The National Strategy for Aging, *2021* aims to expand the scope of LTC by emphasizing home and community-based care, private sector roles, and technology, and the country has also recently published the *Care Economy Roadmap and National Action Plan for a Transformative, Gender-Equal and Just World of Work* in which LTC is a key component.[9]
- **Mongolia**: The National Strategy for Population Ageing (2009–2030) and National Program on Healthy Ageing (2014–2020) aim to enhance older adults' quality of life. The pilot also influenced policy. In 2024, the Elderly Law in Mongolia was revised to incorporate assessment and case management services and increase the budget available for home-based services. As of 2025, the budget for home-based services totaled $1.566 million (MNT5.4 billion) compared with $85,000 (MNT300 million) from previous years.
- **Viet Nam**: The National Strategy on Older Persons Until 2035, With Vision to 2045 approved on 21 February 2025 promote improved health care for older people. The Prime Minister's Decision No. 1648 dated 1 August 2025 aims to establish 12,000 new ISHCs by 2035. There are opportunities to strengthen the policy framework and financing for scaling up the community-based care for older people in the implementation of the revised Health Insurance Law (2024) and the forthcoming National Program on Healthcare, Population, and Development (2026–2035).

---

[9] Government of Indonesia, Ministry of Women's Empowerment and Child Protection. 2024. *Care Economy Roadmap and National Action Plan for a Transformative, Gender-Equal and Just World of Work.*

Rationale for Investing in Community-Based Long-Term Care

Community-based LTC creates a network of care among residents, families, and profit and nonprofit organizations. It aims to improve older people's quality of life. By supporting their aging in place, older adults can remain in familiar environments, which supports mental and emotional well-being. It also fosters independence and autonomy, both of which are crucial for dignity and self-esteem. Community-based LTC also promotes social inclusion and decreases isolation, thereby reducing known risk factors for depression and cognitive decline. It encourages intergenerational interaction and community engagement. Services can be customized to local needs, including language, culture, and tradition.

By supporting their aging in place, older adults can remain in familiar environments, which supports mental and emotional well-being.

Community-based LTC addresses inequities and service disparities by targeting people in greatest need, such as those with low income, and can reach those living in remote rural areas. It is cost-effective and has often been found to be less expensive than residential care in most cases, especially for older people who do not have complex care needs.[10] It also generates cost savings by reducing the burden on public health care systems through prevention of unnecessary hospitalization. There are benefits beyond those for older adults themselves, because community-based LTC services can lead to job creation in caregiving, transportation, and support services. This, in turn, stimulates community-based economies and supports small businesses.

Community-based care also supports family caregivers through respite services and training. This helps prevent caregiver burnout.

[10] L. Di Pollina et al. 2017. Integrated care at home reduces unnecessary hospitalizations of community-dwelling frail older adults: A prospective controlled trial. *BMC Geriatr.* 17 (53); Y. Yi, J. Liu, and L. Jiang. 2023. Does home and community-based services use reduce hospital utilization and hospital expenditure among disabled elders? Evidence from China. *Frontiers in Public Health*; X. Lyu, and Y. Fan. 2024. The Impact of Home- and Community-Based Services on the Health of Older Adults: A Meta-Analysis. *SAGE Open.* 14(3). (Original work published 2024); S. Reinhard et al. 2008. Supporting Family Caregivers in Providing Care. In R. Hughes, ed. Patient Safety and Quality: An Evidence-Based Handbook for Nurses. Agency for Healthcare Research and Quality. April Chapter 14.

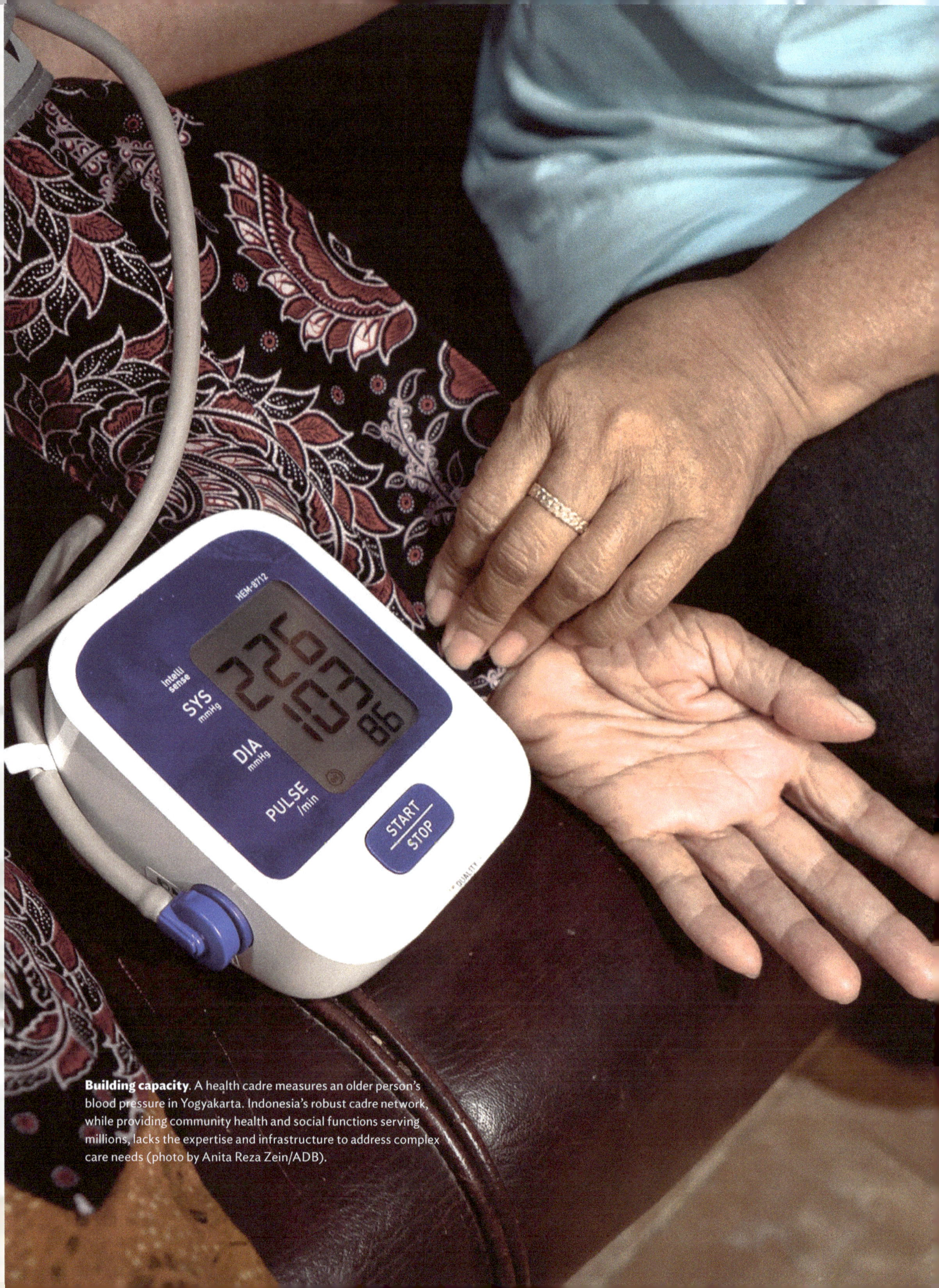

Building capacity. A health cadre measures an older person's blood pressure in Yogyakarta. Indonesia's robust cadre network, while providing community health and social functions serving millions, lacks the expertise and infrastructure to address complex care needs (photo by Anita Reza Zein/ADB).

Regional Pilot to Develop Community-Based Long-Term Care Systems and Services

In December 2019, ADB approved a new regional project, Developing Innovative Community-Based Long-term Care Systems and Services, with financing from the High-Level Technology Fund, the Japan Fund for Prosperous and Resilient Asia and the Pacific, the Japan Special Fund, and the Technical Assistance Special Fund (footnote 2). The project sought to develop innovative and sustainable community-based LTC service models that can operate in low-income settings, deliver quality and affordable services, are sustainable and have potential for replication, build the knowledge base on LTC, and strengthen knowledge sharing and networking on LTC in the region.[11] The project built on the findings, recommendations, and lessons learned of earlier technical assistance, which improved strategic planning and policy development in LTC in the same countries.[12]

In each country, a community-based care pilot project, financed and supported with technical assistance from ADB, was designed through a participatory process.

In each country, a community-based care pilot project, financed and supported with technical assistance from ADB, was designed through a participatory process and based on three key principles:

- support aging in place,
- build on local community assets that link but don't duplicate existing health and social services, and
- provide integrated holistic services that meet the diverse needs of older people and their families.

These principles and the vision—to live longer, healthier, and happier—lay the foundation for a person-centered approach (Table 2). At the heart of the project was a series of community-based LTC pilots, promoting active aging, care and support services, case management, and information referral.

[11] The project originally included Sri Lanka but, due to unforeseen circumstances, did not proceed there.

[12] ADB. 2022. *Technical Assistance Completion Report: Strengthening Developing Member Countries' Capacity in Elderly Care*.

Table 2. Community-Based Long-Term Care Model

	Indonesia	Mongolia	Viet Nam
Mission	To develop innovative and sustainable community-based long-term care service models to operate in low-income settings, delivering quality and affordable services that are sustainable and replicable		
Target Group	Older people	Older people	Frail older people
Process	Case management		
Services	Active aging activities, information and referral, and care and support including home care visits	Access to basic needs and information, rehabilitation, day care, social and educational activities, and home care visits	Home visits, health checks, support in accessing benefits, and mobilization of community and local government resources to meet specific needs
Service Providers	New community care hubs (CCHs): community organizations at the village level	Active aging hubs implemented by existing service providers: general hospital, elder development center, and nongovernment organization	Case management system linking existing health staff with community organizations, overseen by Commune Care Coordinating Committees
Links to Health Services	CCHs linked with government-run community health clinics through appointed senior case managers (*puskesmas*)	Co-located with or outreach to health services	Linked to local health services (commune health stations) through appointed Commune Health Stations case managers

Source: Compiled by authors.

Models of Care

A model of care provides the framework for delivering LTC services. It outlines the principles, the roles of different stakeholders, the key and unique features, the building blocks and the sequence of how they connect, and what can be expected in terms of service outputs and outcomes.[13]

Although the modalities varied between the three countries, programs included information and referral systems, active aging initiatives, and care and support services tailored to older adults.

In pre-project consultations, the stakeholders envisioned a case management system targeting the population of older people. In this overarching care model, high-risk older adults are assessed for biopsychosocial needs by trained case managers before the enhancement and coordination of formal and informal services, such as care and support services by trained paid staff or volunteer caregivers. Lower-risk older adults are engaged with an active aging program, and a less resource-intensive information and referral service.

Three Contexts, Three Models of Care

Each of the three countries conceptualized the pilot slightly differently. In Indonesia, the pilot project comprised five community care hubs (CCHs) at the village level, three in Yogyakarta, and two in Bali. In Mongolia, the project piloted three active aging hubs (AAHs) in Ulaanbaatar, Darkhan-Uul, and Mandal Soum, three settings run by three different types of organizations. In Viet Nam, the focus of the project was 12 village case management teams across four communes, two each in the provinces of Hoa Binh and Thanh Hoa.

The organization of the pilot project varied by country. In Indonesia, it integrated with local village offices. In Mongolia, one pilot project operated as an add-on to a residential care facility, another operated as an independent entity, and a third operated as an extension of a local hospital. In Viet Nam, the pilot project functioned as an outreaching case management team, and integrated with local government and commune health stations.

Although the modalities varied between the three countries, programs included information and referral systems, active aging initiatives, and care and support services tailored to older adults. The care models all embodied three fundamental components: services, a case management system to create individualized care plans and coordination, and overall organizational development and care system integration.

---

[13] H. Vrijhoef. ComSA Evaluation study. Unpublished.

Services

All pilot providers established care hubs or case management teams to deliver active aging, care and support, and information and referral services. All these are basic but essential LTC services. In Viet Nam, as the ISHC network is already a highly successful and sustainable program that runs active aging activities, the pilot project focused on the development of the case management system.

Social engagement, learning, a healthy diet, and regular exercise can help delay age-related conditions like sarcopenia and frailty.

Active aging programs provided activities to encourage social engagement, learning, a healthy diet, and regular exercise. These activities can also help delay age-related conditions like sarcopenia and frailty. In Indonesia and Mongolia, older adults were given access to active aging programs, which promoted leisure, socialization, adult learning, volunteerism, and health promotion. For senior citizens needing a higher level of support, active aging programs were delivered at home through care and support services.

Care and support services were for individuals with specific care requirements and limited family support. They and their caregivers could receive direct assistance with daily living tasks such as homemaking and personal care, including assistance with meals and bathing. These services also included social visits to isolated seniors by neighbors and community volunteers. In Indonesia, cadres actively participated in delivering care and support, as did AAH staff in Mongolia. In Viet Nam, case management teams closely coordinated care and support services with community care volunteers.

Information and referral services helped older adults and caregivers access government and community resources. Some individuals only needed information or connections to other service providers. For example, information and referral services in the Indonesia pilot helped people obtain health insurance cards and social assistance, while in Viet Nam, through case management services, a number of individuals were identified as eligible for disability allowances. Information and referral are an approach to connect services to an individual that is less resource-intensive than the actual case management (see below) which requires a comprehensive needs assessment and customized care plan.

Case Management System

The case management system is a key component of a population health approach and in all three countries aimed to provide integrated care for older people, from the healthy to the frail. A case management system comprises case finding, risk stratification, service matching, and case management (Figure 1).

Case management is defined as "a dynamic process that assesses, plans, implements, coordinates, monitors, and evaluates to improve outcomes, experiences, and value for individuals and families. It is a collaborative effort that involves identifying needs, coordinating services, and advocating for clients' rights and access to support."[14]

---

[14] Definition of "case management" by the American Case Management Association used in the pilot sites.

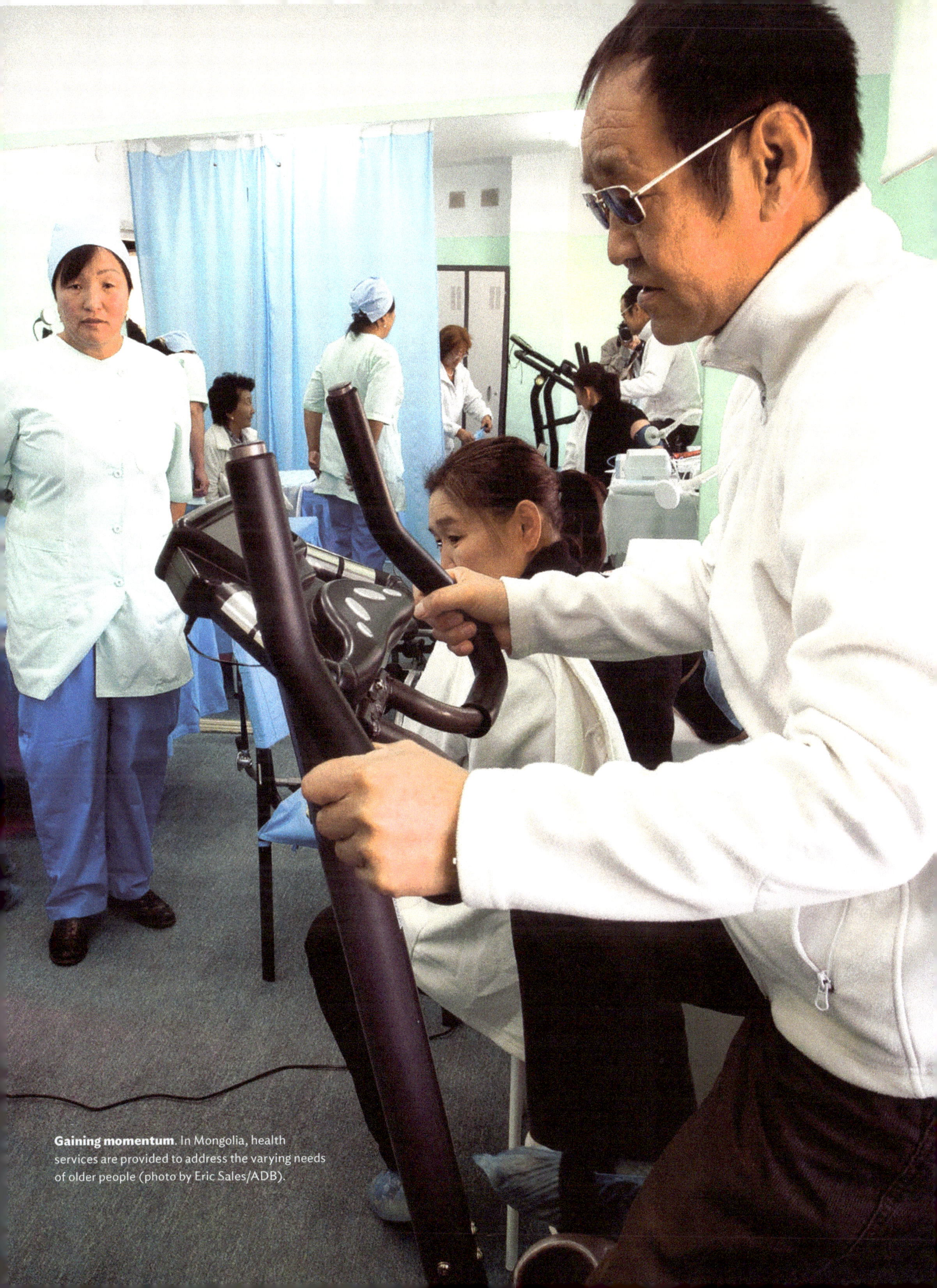

Gaining momentum. In Mongolia, health services are provided to address the varying needs of older people (photo by Eric Sales/ADB).

The key components of a case management service include

- comprehensive needs assessment that triggers 'care foci,' i.e., areas of common LTC health and psychosocial need that would benefit from intervention and support;
- care planning;
- care plan execution and monitoring;
- review of care needs and the care plan;
- documentation and monitoring of the care journey; and
- use of clinical protocols developed to guide the care plans for each of the care foci triggered by the comprehensive needs assessment.

The gatekeeping and stratification process inherent in the case management process ensures resources are efficiently allocated, which, in turn, enhances equity, sustainability, and quality of care.

Figure 1: Case Management Flow

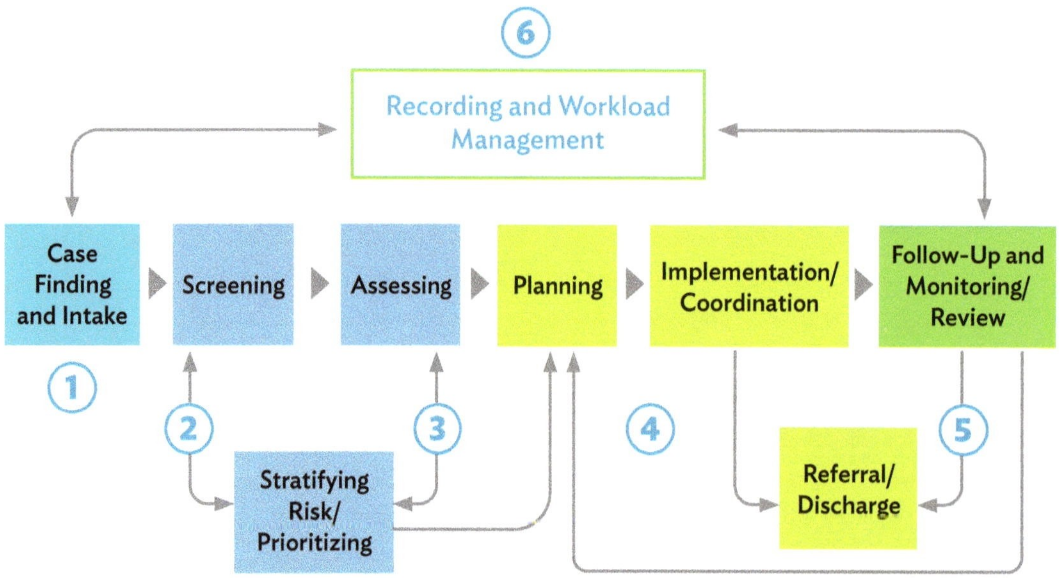

Source: Adapted from the Commission for Case Manager Certification. 2025. Case Management Body of Knowledge.

Case finding can be active, where community workers conduct community-wide door-to-door visits to known seniors, using a standardized tool for risk screening assessment. Passive case finding involves at-risk seniors being referred to the case management service by primary health care services or other community agencies. In Indonesia, the case-finding process used the government's Elderly Information System (SILANI) data collection tool for risk screening, and capturing screening domains like ADLs, IADLs, disability, mood, and cognition (footnote 3). In Mongolia and Viet Nam, the risk screening tool used the Clinical Frailty Scale[15] and a question to confirm the presence of an informal caregiver. This is significant because, if there is an informal caregiver, risk and vulnerability are somewhat reduced.

[15] Dalhousie University. Clinical Frailty Scale.

Risk stratification categorizes older adults into levels of vulnerability based on the risk screening tool's scoring algorithm. The pilot took reference from the Kaiser Permanente Care Pyramid as a gatekeeping framework.[16] This stratifies older adults into three tiers based on risk and care complexity:

Service matching connects older adults to services according to their risk level.

- **Level 1**: Older adults are healthy and require minimal support for both instrumental and regular activities of daily life, but may benefit from active aging activities.
- **Level 2**: Older adults have some health problems that put them at risk of mild or even severe functional impairment. In addition to active aging activities, they may need some formal support.
- **Level 3**: Older adults are vulnerable and frail, with moderate to severe functional impairment. They require a comprehensive needs assessment, care plan, and coordination of services.

Service matching connects older adults to services according to their risk level (Table 3). Older adults categorized as Level 1 or 2 are encouraged to participate in active aging programs. Level 2 older adults receive more frequent risk screening, and some may receive case management services at the case manager's discretion. Level 3 older adults are recommended for case management service.

Table 3: Service Matching Recommendations

Risk Stratification Level	Service/ Resource Matching
Level 1	▪ Active aging, growth and development programs ▪ May be engaged and trained to be volunteers or additional workforce ▪ Receive risk screening at least once every 1 to 2 years
Level 2	▪ Active aging, growth and development programs ▪ Access to formal support may be needed, e.g., information and referral service ▪ Comprehensive needs assessment is generally not needed, unless there is a crisis or under special circumstances at the case managers' discretion ▪ Should receive risk screening at least once every 6 months
Level 3	▪ Care management supported by age-friendly primary health care is needed, i.e., requires a comprehensive needs assessment, a care plan and varying degrees of service navigation and care coordination ▪ Home-based, center-based or residential-based long-term care services may be needed ▪ Active aging, growth and development programs should still be introduced

Source: Compiled by authors.

[16] A. Barceló et al. 2012. *Improving Chronic Illness Care through Integrated Health Service Delivery Networks.* Pan Am Health Organization.

For those categorized at Level 3, and occasionally for those categorized at Level 2, case managers and associate case managers conducted comprehensive needs assessments to develop personalized care plans. These assessments spanned biological, functional, psychological, social, and spiritual dimensions, ensuring that all aspects of the individual's well-being were considered. This holistic approach allowed for the development of care plans that addressed the individual's unique needs and preferences. The comprehensive needs assessment was standardized across the three countries, with only minor differences among them.

The comprehensive needs assessment was standardized across the three countries, with only minor differences among them.

The unique features of this case management system include having clear algorithmic instructions built into the comprehensive needs assessment that trigger the care foci (Table 4). Care foci are areas of regularly occurring care-related need faced by frail elders and their caregivers. There are four categories of care foci that cover the clinical, psycho-emotional, socioeconomic and functional needs of Level 3 older people. The system also included frequent interdisciplinary group meetings between the case management service and the primary health care services, with senior clinical staff from the primary health care service playing a supervisory role in the interdisciplinary team. With such arrangements, the LTC service is designed to be person-centered, holistic, integrated, evidence-informed, and consistent in its delivery of care.

Table 4: Prevalence of Care Foci Among Older Adults Classified as Level 3, with Viet Nam as an Example

Care Foci		Viet Nam (%) March 2025
A. Functional	Challenge in mobility	92.0
	Visual impairment	62.7
	Hearing impairment	56.0
	Communication deficit	56.0
	Basic activities of daily living impairment	82.7
	Instrumental activities of daily living impairment	90.7
	Sarcopenia and fall risk	69.3
B. Psycho-emotional	Cognitive impairment	58.7
	Low mood risk	78.7
	Challenging behavior	12.0
	Loneliness	50.7
	Spiritual needs	29.3
C. Socio-economic	Environmental risk	32.0
	Caregiver stress	49.3
	Elder abuse risk	4.0
	Financial strain	44.0
D. Clinical	Noncommunicable disease	68.0
	Polypharmacy	20.0
	Medication management	14.7
	Dehydration risk	24.0
	Malnourishment risk	61.3
	Sleep problems	66.7
	Loss of appetite	54.7
	Pain	84.0
	Dental problems	64.0
	Wounds, rashes, or itches	18.7
	Cardiorespiratory issues	36.0
	Bowel problems	52.0
	Urinary incontinence	41.3
	Preventive health	78.7
	Advanced care planning	26.7

Source: Compiled by authors.

Case conferences exemplify team-based care by fostering collaboration and coordination among team members and external stakeholders. As part of the case management implementation/coordination processes, case conferences were organized regularly. In 2024, the five CCHs in Indonesia, for example, held up to 15 case conferences per month among them. Case conferences were crucial for multidisciplinary teams to collaborate, share information, and coordinate care plans. In all three countries, these teams typically comprised care professionals such as nurses, social workers, and physicians, as well as nonprofessional workers such as associate case managers, active aging programmers, care aides, and volunteers. Case conferences enabled teams to discuss the progress of individual care plans, identify and address challenges or concerns, adjust care plans to meet the evolving needs of older adults, and ensure seamless transitions between care settings or providers. At these meetings, senior case managers, who could be physicians, nurses, or social workers, provided clinical guidance and linkages to upstream social and health care providers, such as hospitals and rehabilitation centers.

Case conferences were crucial for multidisciplinary teams to collaborate, share information, and coordinate care plans.

Community asset mapping and coordination with other community organizations enhanced home and community-based care development in Indonesia, Mongolia, and Viet Nam by leveraging local resources and fostering collaborative networks. In each country, the community asset mapping identified local government resources (such as social assistance programs and transport services), community organizations and NGOs, and private companies and individuals willing to provide time and resources to support older people. These strategies of engaging people and neighborhood assets empower communities, optimize resources, and created scalable, culturally relevant home care models across these three countries.

Overall Organizational Development and Care System Integration

The project introduced system management, starting with the development of strategic, business, and functional plans for specific teams. This included prototypes for CCHs in Indonesia and AAHs in Mongolia. These plans, along with operational and program manuals, covered various aspects of hub and team management, such as financing, staffing, quality and risk management, and networking.

Indonesia's Service Delivery Model

There are limited LTC services in Indonesia and they are highly fragmented. The pilot project sought to address this by developing CCHs, where older adults and their caregivers could be connected to the services they needed, and those services could operate in a more coordinated manner. The care model promotes both horizontal and vertical integration, encompassing district health centers (*Pusat Kesehatan Masyarakat* or *puskesmas*); hospitals;medical specialists; private sector involvement; and community-based assets/resources, such as women's groups (*Pemberdayaan dan Kesejahteraan Keluarga*), community groups (*Bina Keluarga Lansia*), and health stations (*Posyandu Lansia*).

Community-based LTC services were delivered through five CCHs at the village level (Figure 2), with case management and a digital information system as key system facilitators to coordinate three care hubs in Yogyakarta (Banyuraden, Guwosari, and Wirogunan) and two in Bali (Pedungan and Melinggih). These hubs were typically organized within village offices, which provided space for their operations and service delivery. The CCHs in Indonesia strived to offer services not readily available in the community, such as care and support. They served as central points of information and referral. Over time, existing active elder care programs were aligned with the activities conducted by the CCHs. Also, the CCHs developed new and innovative active aging initiatives.

These hubs aimed to integrate information and referrals, active aging, care and support (e.g., home help and home care), and respite care under a single administrative umbrella. The hubs also linked older adults with LTC needs with a network of care, such as primary care providers, nurse-based elder centers, community health stations, social centers, elder and family education groups, and women's groups. This integration through case management streamlined service delivery, making it more efficient and accessible for older adults.

Figure 2: Indonesia's Community Care Hub Model

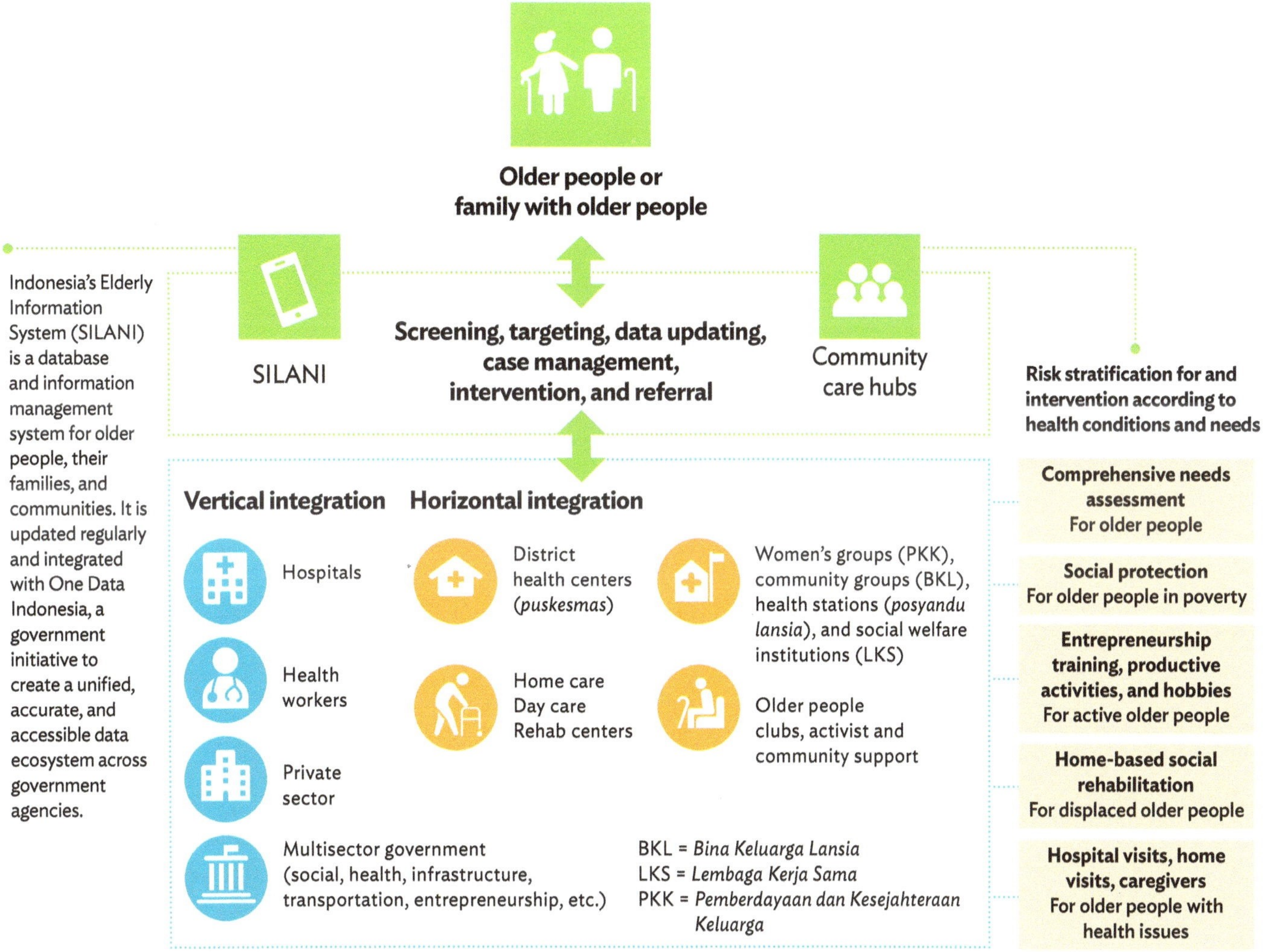

Source: Results of Community-Based Mapping and Assessment conducted with ADB support.

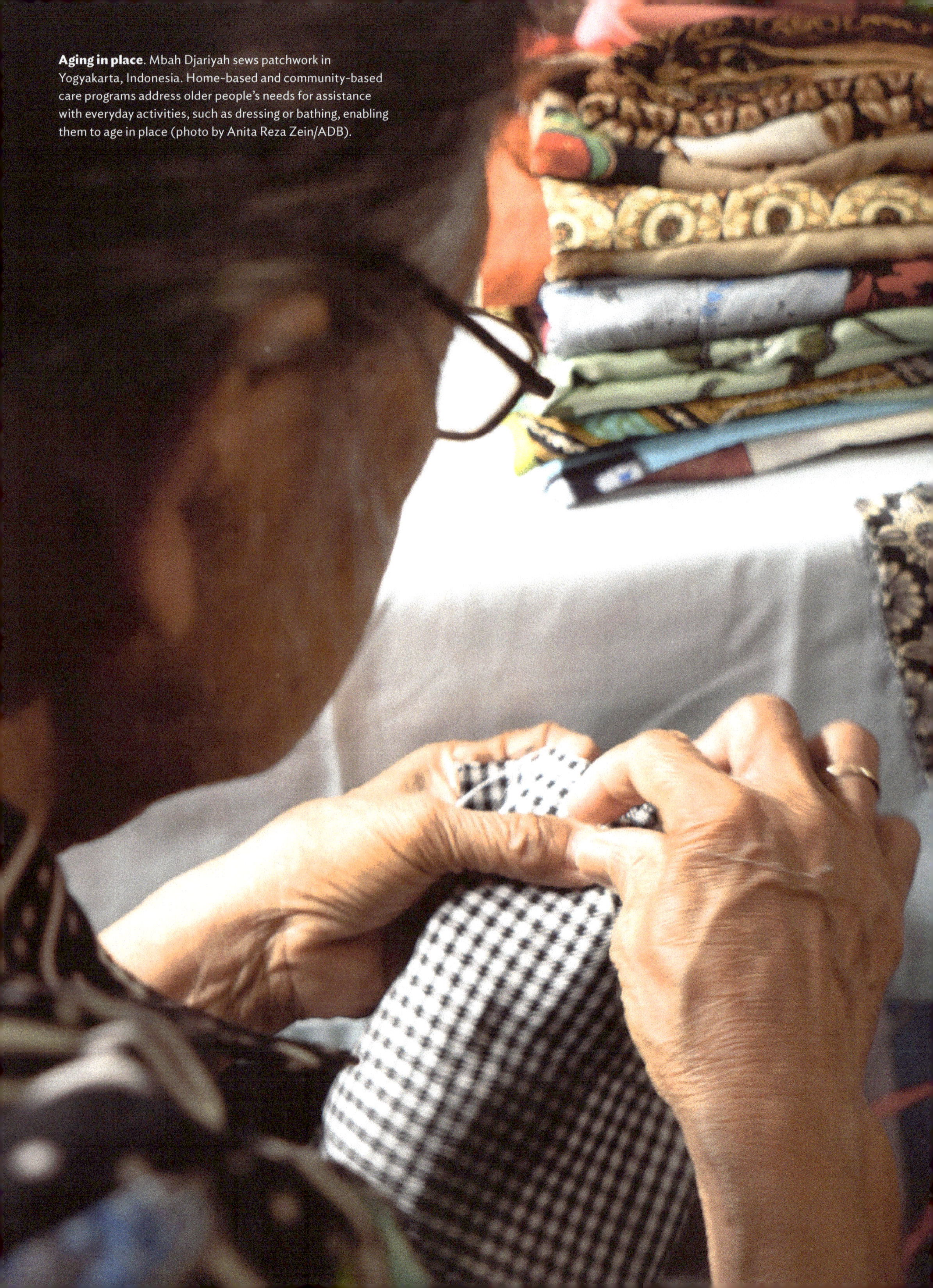

Aging in place. Mbah Djariyah sews patchwork in Yogyakarta, Indonesia. Home-based and community-based care programs address older people's needs for assistance with everyday activities, such as dressing or bathing, enabling them to age in place (photo by Anita Reza Zein/ADB).

The CCHs operated under the authority of the village government, making all hub activities an integral part of the responsibilities of the village head. The CCHs also collaborated with the local health center (*puskesmas*), civil society organizations, and other community-based institutions including ambulance operators and related government agencies, to ensure support for its activities and services. This collaborative structure fostered community engagement, aligned the hub's activities with local needs, and leveraged the expertise of various stakeholders to efficiently deliver essential services. In the future, an advisory board or committee will be appointed by the village head, and be responsible for providing direction, guidance, supervision, and support to the CCH.

Community care hubs collaborated with the local health center, civil society organizations, and other community-based institutions including ambulance operators and related government agencies.

The daily operation of each hub was overseen by an operations manager, who served as the business lead, supported by a case manager. The operations manager was responsible for strategic planning, developing the business plan, and organizing the CCH. This included securing resources, managing daily operations, and coordinating active aging activities with the assistance of the active aging programmer. The case manager oversaw case management, care, and support.

The hub's operations benefited from diverse support sources, ensuring sustainability and community engagement. Initial funding from ADB covered equipment requirements and care hub staff honoraria, while village offices provided complimentary space and administrative support. Local communities contributed through cash and in-kind donations. On the cessation of the pilot, funding for hub activities and staff was secured from a variety of sources depending on locality, including village funds and municipalities, through social welfare, and via family planning offices, supplemented by local fundraising and donations. Maintaining the value of the honoraria for CCH staff also depended on local regulations and funding mechanisms. As most of the costs involved in care are related to human resources, ensuring a reliable funding source to adequately compensate CCH staff is a key future priority.

Local governments in Yogyakarta and Bali have started to expand CCHs to other communities, mobilizing local financing and providing coordinated training and mentoring.

Mongolia's Service Delivery Model

Mongolia's LTC services are provided by a range of providers, with a heavy emphasis on medical-based care. The pilot sought to develop an AAH model with three types of providers, across three geographical settings.

There were three AAHs in the Mongolia pilot project (Figure 3). One was run by Achlalt Khuukhduud, an NGO in Songinokhairkhan district, Ulaanbaatar (district population 343,000). A second was housed in the government-run Elderly Development Centre in Darkhan-Uul *aimag* (province) (population 100,000), and a third in the general hospital in Mandal Soum of Selenge *aimag* (population 27,000). The hubs promoted active and healthy aging through a wide range of activities, including physical exercise, rehabilitation, nutritional awareness, public health training, capacity building and empowerment, stress management, communication technology skills, volunteering, and economic productive activities. These hubs also brought together information and referrals, home help and outreach services, and adult day care under one administration.

Figure 3: Active Aging Hub Model

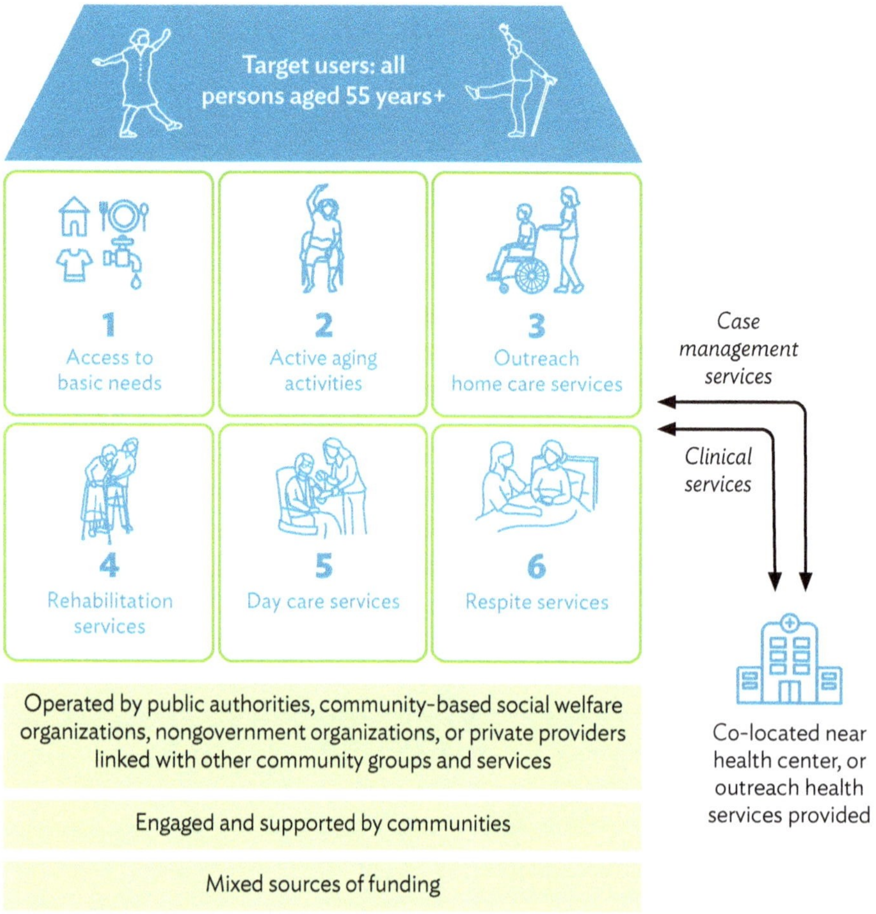

Source: Authors.

Achlalt Khuukhduud was a provider of residential care, home care, and adult day care for older people and people with disabilities. During the pilot, as an AAH provider, the organization collaborated closely with local community organizations such as family care centers, elder associations, and government agencies. These organizations adhered to a case management process with clear roles and responsibilities. Achlalt Khuukhduud was responsible for caring for older adults categorized at Level 3, the primary care center served older people categorized at Level 2, and the elder association supported those categorized at Level 1.

In Darkhan-Uul *aimag*, the AAH was a stand-alone hub that was originally designed as an elder development center. It adopted case management and offered a comprehensive range of elder care services under one roof, including primary care, rehabilitation, and active aging programs that focused on social and recreational activities. During the pilot, the center provided outreach case management services for Level 3 older adults, and coordinated with social workers, family health doctors, and Red Cross volunteers.

In Mandal Soum, the AAH was integrated into a general hospital. It offered active aging activities, care and support as part of its outpatient services, provided outreach case management to individuals at Levels 2 and 3 (Figure 4), and coordination with *bagh*[17] family health doctors and social workers. These services were enhanced with the mobilization of community assets and resources. Case management was used to connect service providers and to link older adults in need with volunteers with the necessary skills.

Case management was used to connect service providers and to link older adults in need with volunteers with the necessary skills.

The AAH project in Mongolia was overseen by a national steering committee, chaired by a director of the Population and Development Department in the Ministry of Family, Labour and Social Protection. This committee comprised members of various ministries and agencies, including health, finance, social insurance, and social welfare as well as representatives of the *aimag* and the National Gerontology Centre and Elderly Association. The committee played a crucial role in supporting and guiding the development of LTC initiatives in the country. A local steering committee focused on the planning, operation, and monitoring of each of the AAHs. This committee mirrored the national committee structure.

During the pilot implementation, all three AAH providers funded human resources and activities from their existing resources. Mongolia's AAHs deployed diverse funding models. Darkhan-Uul *aimag*'s Elderly Development Centre, fully funded by the local government, leveraged substantial resources to support AAH operations, redirecting staffing and operational costs. Mandal Soum as a general hospital sustained its AAH by reallocating revenue from the hospital. Achlalt Khuukhduud operated with mixed funding sources from contracted services and fundraising.

Viet Nam's Service Delivery Model

Viet Nam has an extensive network of Intergenerational Self-Help Clubs (ISHCs), and a strong volunteer culture in its services for older adults. The pilot aimed to better connect these existing networks and resources to the medical system, so that older adults could be better served in both their health and social needs.

Viet Nam's LTC model (Figure 4) employed case management teams in 12 villages across Thanh Hoa and Hoa Binh provinces.

[17] A *bagh* is a sub-*soum* administrative unit. A *soum* is a sub-province administrative unit.

Figure 4. Stakeholder Mapping and Structure of Viet Nam's Care Model

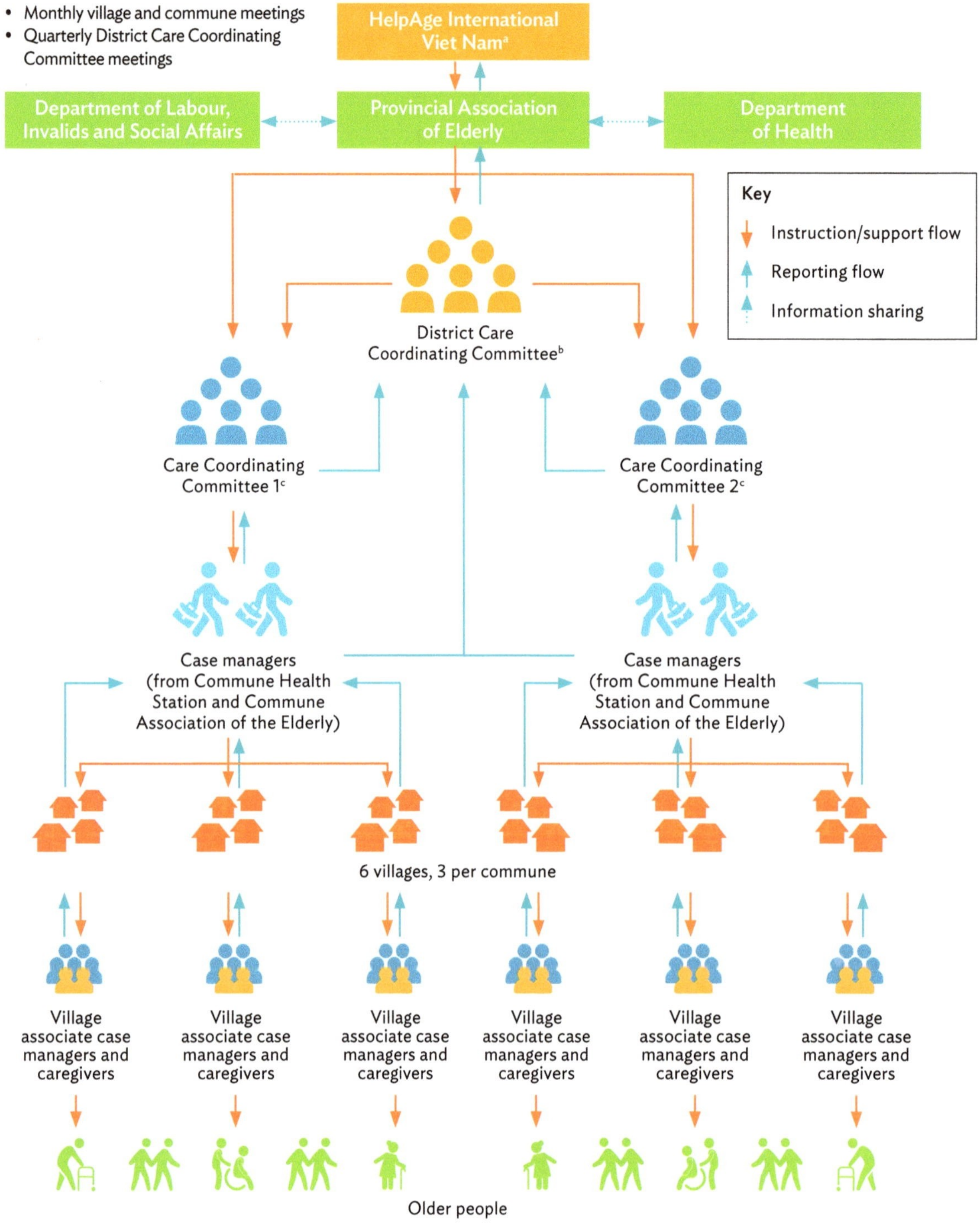

Notes:

[a] HelpAge International Viet Nam was engaged under the technical assistance to support the implementation of the community-based care pilot in the country.

[b] Comprises District People's Committee; District Association of Elderly; District Health Center; Department of Labour, Invalids and Social Affairs; Fatherland Front; and others. The District Care Coordinating Committee is headed by the Vice Chair of the District People's Committee. However, these district-level entities were abolished by the government in July 2025.

[c] Comprises Commune People's Committee; Commune Association of Elderly; Commune Health Center; Social Affairs Officer; Fatherland Front; and others. The Commune Care Coordinating Committee is headed by the Vice Chair of the Commune People's Committee.

Sources: Country Presentation - Viet Nam, Regional Conference on Community-Based Care Models: Learning from DMC Experience. Centara Riverside Hotel, Chiang Mai, Thailand. 28 November–1 December 2023.

Each village-level team comprised two associate case managers, and five trained care volunteers (caregivers). The village-level teams were supported at the commune level by two case managers, a staff member (nurse or medical doctor) from the commune health station, and a social worker from the local elder association. There were clear reporting and supporting relationships between case managers, associate case managers, and care volunteers. Notably, all associate case managers and volunteers came from the village in which they worked. These teams were able to efficiently and effectively use available community resources, particularly care volunteers and donations. The case management teams conducted regular visits to risk-screen all older people in their respective villages, although they were only able to provide care and support to a limited number of Level 3 older people, usually about five per village.

In Viet Nam, case management teams were overseen by the following:

- In each district, a district community care coordinating committee, led by the District People's Committee vice chair, comprising representatives from health, labor, and social affairs. Its primary function was to provide guidance on management of care provision to older people and to identify the necessary resources for the case management team.
- In each commune, commune community care coordinating committees, headed by the Commune Peoples' Committee vice chair, responsible for ensuring the quality and standards of care at the commune level and troubleshooting.
- In each village, the case management was facilitated by case managers and associate case managers by bringing together community caregivers and local leaders. Their primary focus was on reviewing care plans, troubleshooting. and facilitating skill-sharing among members.

The integration of health and social care was exemplified by the collaborative efforts of the case management teams, local health stations, and the elder associations. The case management teams, comprising representatives of both organizations, worked together to identify and support older people at risk. This model demonstrated social and care integration, fostering collaboration between agencies and community groups to provide cohesive support for timely response to the needs of older people in the community.

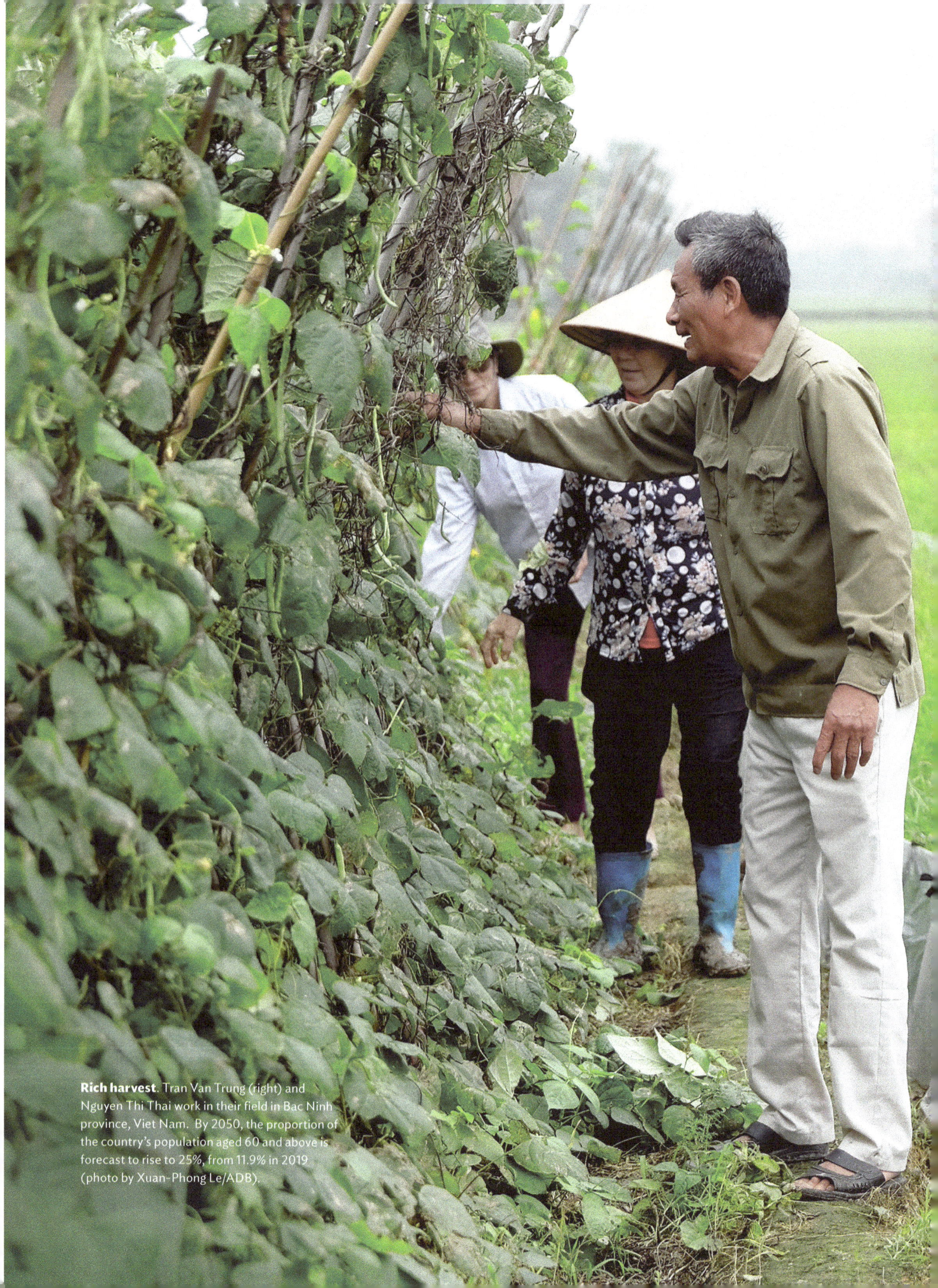

Rich harvest. Tran Van Trung (right) and Nguyen Thi Thai work in their field in Bac Ninh province, Viet Nam. By 2050, the proportion of the country's population aged 60 and above is forecast to rise to 25%, from 11.9% in 2019 (photo by Xuan-Phong Le/ADB).

Community-Based Long-Term Care Workforce

A robust and skilled workforce is essential for an effective community-based LTC system. Besides direct professional and nonprofessional care workers, team leaders and administrators, family caregivers, and volunteer corps play an instrumental role. Capacity building, not only for professional stakeholders but also for family caregivers and volunteers, is key to strengthening the community-based LTC workforce. This section examines the role of professional staff, family caregivers and volunteers, and what was learned from the pilot about these groups. It then describes the pilot's capacity-building elements, including curriculum development and the training modules applied to different stakeholder groups.

A robust and skilled workforce is essential for an effective community-based long-term care system.

Management, Health, and Social Care Workforce

Community care workers, who also serve as assistant case managers (or associate case managers), are responsible for some case management activities, such as screening and implementing care plans, including providing care and support.

Nurses and social workers, who also serve as case managers or senior case managers, are professionally responsible for overall case management. They supervise assistant case managers (or associate case managers) and, when required, perform duties appropriate to the scope of nursing or social work practice.

Senior case managers, who are nurses or physicians at community health centers (Indonesia) or on the staff of an AAH (Mongolia), supervise junior case management staff and serve as a linkage to the larger health and social care system.

In Indonesia, the CCH identified two further necessary roles:

- **Operations managers**, who manage and secure the necessary resources for the hub and team.
- **Active aging programmers**, who manage active aging activities and build an active aging community.

Other stakeholders—such as the rest of the health care workers in the community health center (Indonesia, Mongolia), elder associations (Mongolia, Viet Nam), and representatives of civil society and government—are all critical in the integration of the care, quality management, and development of the program.

What the Pilot Found

Professional and management staff are crucial to ensure reliable, replicable, and high-quality care, complementing the contributions of volunteers. The deployment of paid professionals and management staff enabled the pilot projects to handle complex cases, beyond the capacity of volunteers; improve the practices to provide integrated services; and provide important training and mentoring to volunteers, to boost care quality. A common challenge was the workload of the professional staff, with tasks often added to their existing roles. To achieve service coverage to meet the demand, dedicated roles need to be developed.

Indispensable Role of Family Caregivers

Family caregivers are crucial for providing support and assistance to older adults and are the main providers of care to older adults.

What the Pilot Found

Recognizing the demands on family caregivers is vital for sustainable LTC systems, and these caregivers can be supported in four ways:

- respite care offers temporary relief from caregiving duties, allowing family caregivers to rest and take on other responsibilities;
- training and education equip family caregivers with the necessary skills and knowledge for quality care;
- support groups enable family caregivers to connect, share experiences, and access emotional support; and
- in-kind and cash assistance recognize the financial cost of caregiving.

While the pilot projects provided much-appreciated support to family caregivers through respite care, support in accessing services, assistance in providing personal care, and training and education, more needs to be done. An increase in the provision of home care and community care services, to provide additional respite care, is a priority.

In some cases—where there were no family members, or family members were unable to provide adequate and safe care due to their own circumstances or due to the complexity of care needs—options for residential care placement may have been more suitable. However, there is a shortage of available residential care in each of the three countries.

Some families declined the offer of assistance, perhaps reflecting social and cultural norms around caregiving.

Volunteers Are a Valuable Asset

Beyond family, volunteers are often the first point of contact for older adults and their families. Volunteers play multiple roles in community LTC, including

- providing social support, offering companionship, social and recreational activities, and reducing social isolation;
- providing homemaking and personal care services such as assisting in exercise;
- delivering practical assistance, such as food and clothing;
- arranging transportation services;
- facilitating community health and active case finding;
- organizing active aging activities;
- helping with house repair and modification; and
- promoting community engagement, and fostering a sense of community ownership and responsibility for elder care.

What the Pilot Found

Volunteers are well-placed to be engaged in the organization and delivery of a range of active aging programs, and mobilizing community members with specific expertise, interests, and skills to share their passions with others. As many of the volunteers are older people themselves, this is a win–win in active aging. Through the community asset mapping process a number of volunteers were found, who were willing and able to provide specific areas of support, for example in providing transport services and home modifications.

Making optimal use of a volunteer network requires an effective volunteer management system to recruit and screen suitable volunteers with the necessary skills and attributes. These volunteers need clear job descriptions and skills classification, as well as training and orientation to provide them with the knowledge and skills for effective performance. Proper training enables volunteers to collaborate with professionals in complex care scenarios, acting as an additional set of eyes and ears. Additional training is crucial for managing challenging situations such as dementia, stroke, or bedridden individuals. Training guidelines should also be developed for various levels of volunteer, including certification and registration. The volunteer management system is also responsible for monitoring and supervision, and offering guidance, support, and recognition to volunteers. However, the pilot found that there is a need for caregivers from the community to be financially compensated.

Capacity Building

Capacity building is essential for strengthening the community-based LTC workforce. In the pilot, there was a strong emphasis on training and capacity building for everyone involved in LTC management and delivery. The main beneficiaries of capacity-building activities included the pilot operating staff and volunteers, and primary care providers, i.e., *puskesmas* nurses in Indonesia; nurses and social workers from local health stations, geriatricians, and primary care doctors in Mongolia; and elder associations in Viet Nam. Volunteers were also trained on roles, responsibilities, communication skills, and providing appropriate support to older adults. Other beneficiaries included local leaders, government officials, and local elder care providers.

Curriculum Development and Delivery

Core Training Modules

In each country numerous training programs were adapted or developed (Table 5). The training modules were also specifically targeted to the roles of the stakeholder groups of community-based LTC workforce highlighted above. For example, all stakeholders had to undergo training in the basics of LTC, while only the case managers and senior case managers needed to receive in-depth training on how to conduct a comprehensive needs assessment.

All training combined theoretical knowledge with practical application, often using learning collaboratives, i.e., in a plan–do–study–act cycle. Operational and program manuals were developed based on training. A vital component of the capacity-building program was follow-up mentoring sessions, especially on case management when the trainees would share real-life cases and care plans. These were important to assess accurate use of the assessment and tools, as well as build the confidence of those involved in case management.

Trainees also benefited from benchmarking, with project teams visiting and learning from each other. These visits boosted morale and facilitated the sharing of solutions. Indonesian providers and government officials also participated in a community case management benchmarking visit in Singapore, at the invitation of the Tsao Foundation.

Table 5. Training Programs Developed

Country	Training Program	Recommended Duration (no. of hours)
Indonesia	Introduction to long-term care (LTC)	1.5
	Community care hub operations	12
	Case management	15
	Multidisciplinary teamwork and communication	3
	Common LTC conditions	5
	Case management team mentoring	12
	Office manager mentoring	12
Mongolia	Strategic and business planning for active aging hubs	16
	Case management	23
	Establishing outreach services	8
	Establishing informational and referral services	8
Viet Nam	Case management	35
	Caregiving for older people	21
	Common LTC conditions	15
	Case management team mentoring	21

Source: Unpublished reports, technical assistance Developing Innovative Community-Based Long-Term Care Systems and Services (TA 9928).

As a result of the training programs in each country, the program and operational manuals for each pilot project were developed, tested, and refined over the pilot period:

- Mongolia Active Aging Hub Operational and Program Manual;
- Indonesia Operational Manual and Program Manual; and
- Viet Nam Guideline on the Implementation of Case Management System, Guideline on the Clinical Community-based Care for Older Adults, and Guideline on Health Monitoring for Older People.

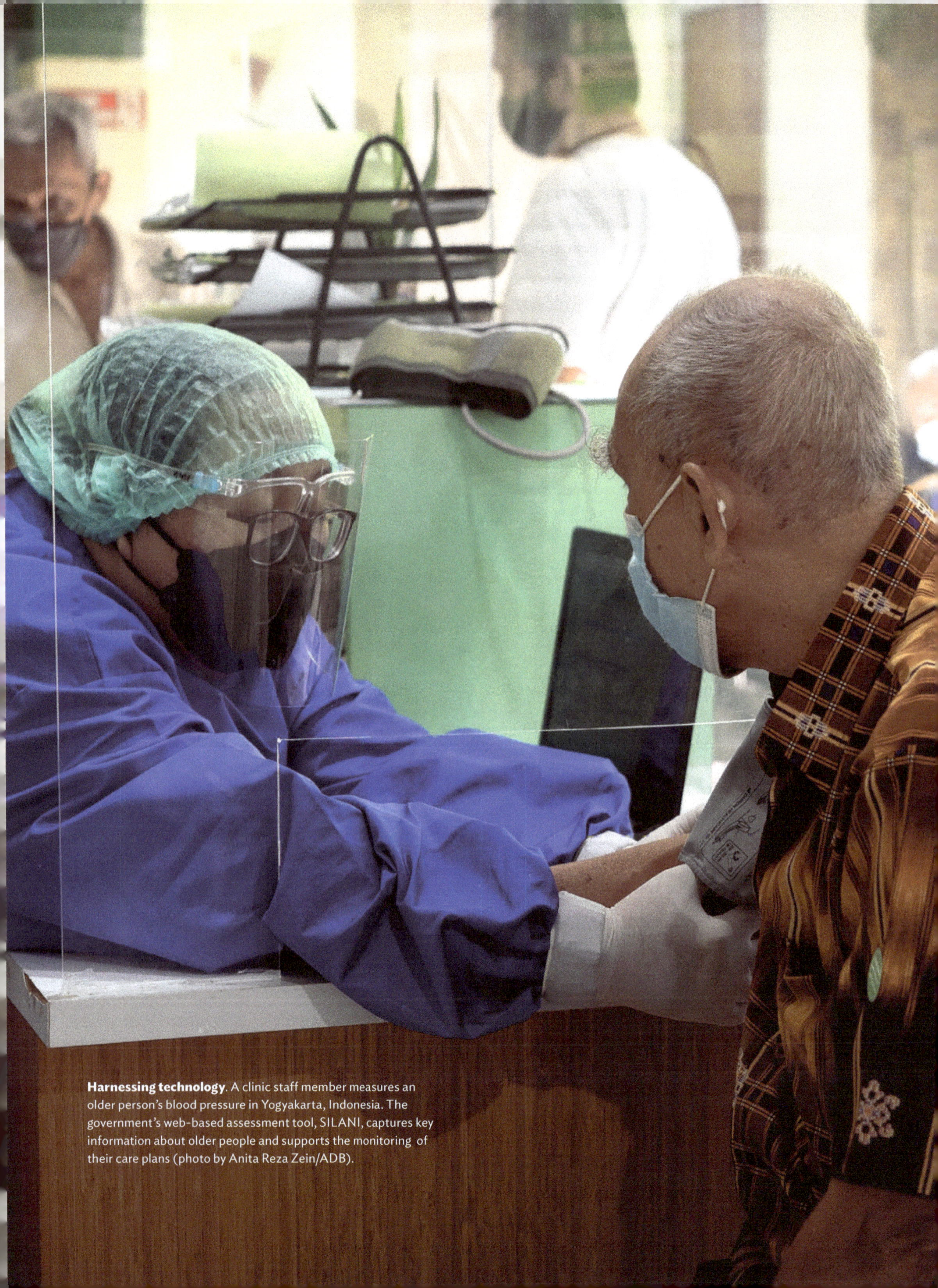

Harnessing technology. A clinic staff member measures an older person's blood pressure in Yogyakarta, Indonesia. The government's web-based assessment tool, SILANI, captures key information about older people and supports the monitoring of their care plans (photo by Anita Reza Zein/ADB).

Innovation and Technology in Long-Term Care in the Pilot

Technology is playing an increasingly vital role in transforming LTC by improving service delivery and coordination. This section examines the pilot's approach to digital care solutions, assistive technology, online care, and data utilization for service planning and policymaking.

Technology is playing an increasingly vital role in transforming long-term care by improving service delivery and coordination.

Digital Care and Case Management

Digital platforms are enhancing communication, care planning, and service delivery in LTC. In Indonesia, the government, through the Ministry of National Development Planning, initiated the web-based assessment tool, SILANI, to survey the health and social status of community-dwelling seniors. SILANI, also available as a mobile app, captures biopsychosocial data, poverty status, caregiver information, seniors' perceived needs, and the geolocation of service providers. The project expanded SILANI into a digital platform for documenting and monitoring Level 3 older adults, incorporating the comprehensive needs assessment, care-foci-triggering algorithm, and digital care plan.

Case management systems are crucial for coordinating care for older adults with complex needs by centralizing information and improving communication among providers, social workers, and families. These systems support care plan monitoring, track progress, and issue identification. Mongolia is just starting to digitalize case management system implementation with a mobile application featuring a risk screening tool, comprehensive needs assessment, care-foci-triggering algorithm, and care plan. But practical challenges remain such as gaps in rural connectivity because of intermittent internet connection (e.g., pilot village in Pedungan, Bali), as well as low digital literacy among older adults (e.g., only 20% in Viet Nam's pilot projects used app-based referrals). Some mitigation strategies that can be adopted include offline data synchronization and community digital literacy workshops.

Data Utilization

Technology, especially digitalized case management, facilitates robust data collection, enabling organizations and governments to better understand the needs of older individuals and develop tailored care plans and policies. Data on health conditions, functional limitations, and service utilization helps identify trends, enables efficient resource allocation, and supports evaluation. Data also informs the development of evidence-based practices and guidelines. For example, data on care foci prevalence among older adults classified as Level 3 in Viet Nam highlights vital long-term social and health care needs. When data are routinely collected on an age- and sex-disaggregated basis, it can support better targeting of resources and deeper understanding of their impact on men and women, and different age groups.

Health and Social Care Integration

Integrated care is a person-centered approach that prioritizes the coordination and collaboration of various services to address the complex and multifaceted needs of older adults. It recognizes that health and social factors are inextricably linked, and that effective care requires a comprehensive strategy. This paradigm breaks down the traditional barriers between health care providers, social service agencies, and community organizations, to promote a seamless continuum of care.

Integrated care recognizes that health and social factors are inextricably linked, and that effective care requires a comprehensive strategy.

The case management system affects care integration, both horizontally—whereby community health and social services are activated and coordinated to meet the special and specific needs of the older people and their caregivers—and vertically, when the older people transit seamlessly across care settings, particularly between the hospitals and the community (Figure 5). For vertical integration, there were many examples of how case managers discovered serious undiagnosed health issues and injuries during their initial comprehensive needs assessment and, in Indonesia and Mongolia, referred seniors to hospitals, and helped smooth the discharge process for older adults, especially those who lived alone.

Connecting to the Larger Ecosystem

The hub model, as piloted in Indonesia and Mongolia, exemplifies integration, capitalizing on existing community assets to support older adults. Different parties each play key roles: local governments provide oversight and accountability, promote coordination, and mobilize resources; NGOs offer essential support services and advocacy; educational institutions train professionals; and community groups provide invaluable social support and combat isolation.

The organization of case management teams in Viet Nam exemplifies this collaborative approach, with health station and elder association case managers, associate case managers, and volunteer caregivers working together. The Commune Care Coordinating Committees ensure quality, risk management, monitoring, and resourcing.

Community-based LTC encompasses more than just health and social needs. Partnerships with diverse sectors—including transportation, housing, and technology—are essential for creating a seamless continuum of care. Partnerships with the private sector bring innovation and resources. A coordinated approach fosters resource sharing, service delivery, and policy development. A central coordinating body can oversee LTC services, ensuring consistent, person-centered care. The pilot model can be integrated with the World Health Organization (WHO) Guidelines on Integrated Care for Older People (ICOPE) approach (Box 2).

Figure 5: How Integrated Care Is Achieved Through Case Management

Sareng, an 87-year-old from Bali, was categorized as Level 3 using SILANI, the Risk Screening and Risk Stratification Tool. As a result, she was enrolled into the case management service. The Comprehensive Needs Assessment identified the following care foci:

Cognitive and psychological

1. Cognitive impairment
2. Loneliness

Clinical

1. Untreated hypertension because Sareng has difficulty attending community health center
2. Back pain

Functional performance

1. Inaccessible environment
2. Unable to walk
3. Unable to go to the toilet
4. Needs help from caregiver in all activities of daily living except eating

Socioeconomic

1. Caregiver is stressed
2. Financial strain

Care Plan Implementation

Cognitive and psychological:

- Sareng receives visits from volunteers in the village.

Clinical:

- Sareng receives home visits from health center nurse.
- Nurse begins Sareng's hypertension treatment under doctor's instruction.
- Sareng is prescribed painkillers.

Functional performance:

- Sareng receives donated diapers and a wheelchair.

Socioeconomic:

- Caregiver receives training on care of person with cognitive impairment.
- Sareng obtains financial aid from social welfare agency.

Outcomes:

- Sareng is less lonely.
- Her hypertension is under control.
- Her pain is reduced.
- The caregiver's stress is reduced.

Next Objective of Care

To organize transport so Sareng can participate in active aging activities in the village community care hub.

* Level 3 older adults are vulnerable and frail, with moderate to severe functional impairment. They require a comprehensive needs assessment, care plan, and coordination of services.

Source: Compiled by authors.

Box 2: World Health Organization ICOPE Approach

Noting the central role of integrated care for older people in 2017, the World Health Organization (WHO) published the WHO Guidelines on Integrated Care for Older People (ICOPE).[a] These propose evidence-based recommendations for health care professionals to prevent, slow, or reverse declines in the physical and mental capacities of older people.[b]

There are four steps in the implementation of ICOPE.[c] Step 1 involves a set of simple binary questions and physical tests to assess for the presence of the six intrinsic capacity deficits. Step 2 involves those screened positively being referred to their primary care providers for confirmation and further in-depth assessment. Step 3 entails the development, implementation, and monitoring of a care plan through a multidisciplinary team across the health and social sectors, with links to local geriatric care services, while Step 4 is the engagement of communities and supporting caregivers.

It is clear that, for ICOPE to achieve its intended objectives, there must be sufficient capacity within the existing primary health care systems for follow-up of all seniors with intrinsic capacity deficits detected, providing sufficient in-depth assessment and coordinating community resources to provide the necessary interventions. Because the main target population for the pilot was older adults who were frail and in need for long-term care services, a different approach was taken, whereby seniors who were already dependent were identified (i.e., classified as Level 3[d]) and matched with a case manager, who, in turn, would provide in-depth assessment and develop an individualized care plan, in close collaboration with the primary health care system.

However, going up-stream to prevent care dependency was very much an objective of the pilot. Thus, if the participating health systems wish to combine ICOPE with this care model, older adults at lower risk levels may still be assessed according to the ICOPE guidelines, starting with Step 1 (Figure a).

[a] WHO. 2017. *Integrated care for older people: guidelines on community-level interventions to manage declines in intrinsic capacity.*

[b] WHO. 2019. *Integrated care for older people: guidance for person-centred assessment and pathways in primary care.*

[c] WHO. 2024. *Integrated care for older people (ICOPE): guidance for person-centred assessment and pathways in primary care.* Second edition.

[d] Level 3 comprises older adults who are vulnerable and frail, with moderate to severe functional impairment. They require a comprehensive needs assessment, care plan, and coordination of services.

Source: Authors.

Figure 6: Combining the ICOPE Approach with Pilot Care Model

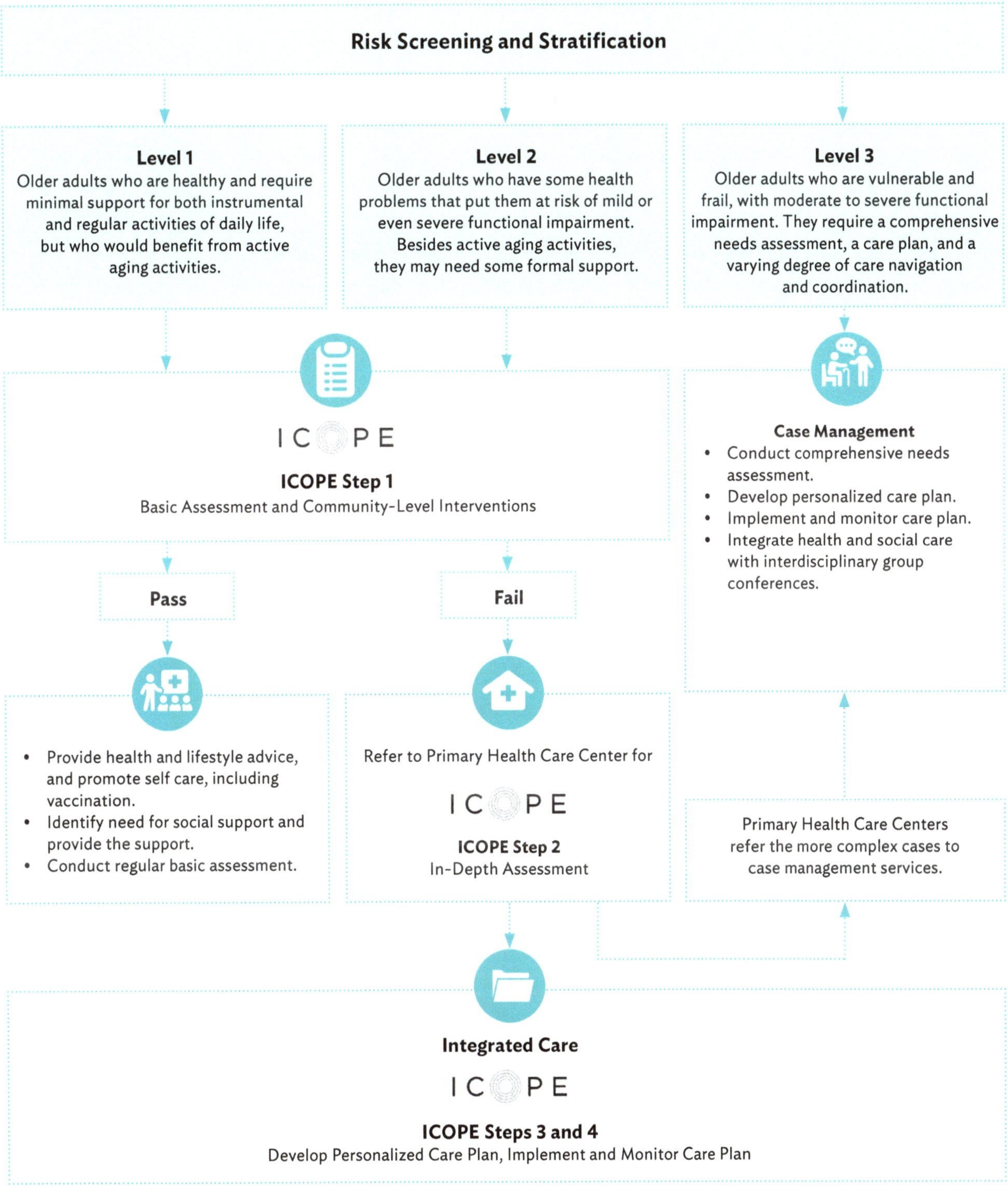

ICOPE = Integrated Care for Older People.
Source: Authors.

Key Successes

The pilot projects reported improved health and social outcomes for older adults, resulting from the provision of care, enhanced access to health care, social assistance and social services, and improved social bonds.

Establishment of innovative community-based LTC system and models. The three models delivered active aging programs, care and support services, as well as information and referral services supported by a robust case management system to support aging in place, through development of home and community-based care services.

Positive impact on older adults and their families. The pilot projects suggest potential benefits for improving health and social outcomes for older adults. These benefits are resulting from enhanced access to health care, social assistance and social services, and improved social bonds. Families experienced reduced caregiving stress through respite care, training, and strengthened emotional bonds.

Population risk screening and stratification. This provided a robust, evidence-based mechanism to target resources efficiently. Thus, care services were prioritized for those who needed them most, preventing over-servicing, and promoting early intervention. In Indonesia, the SILANI tool facilitated risk screening, while Mongolia and Viet Nam used internationally recognized tools such as the Clinical Frailty Scale.

Effective case management systems. Individualized care plans, using the care foci framework, ensured holistic responses, particularly for frail older adults. Regular case conferences involving multidisciplinary teams, enhanced coordination, health and social integration, and care quality.

Coordination of health and social care services. In Indonesia, CCHs linked with *puskesmas*, hospitals, and community groups. Mongolia's AAHs collaborated with primary care centers, social workers and elder associations. Viet Nam's case management teams partnered with commune health stations and the elder associations. This integration ensured cohesive support, addressing both medical and psychosocial needs, and fostered multisector partnerships with local governments and NGOs.

Strong support from local and national authorities. The robust support provided by national and local authorities in all three countries was pivotal to the success of the pilot projects. Each country seamlessly integrated pilot projects into existing institutions (e.g., village offices in Indonesia, commune health stations in Viet Nam); and aligned the projects with national strategies related to aging and LTC. Their unwavering commitment ensured relevance and ownership, establishing the foundation of a national-scale expansion of these innovative care models.

Changes in attitudes and understanding. Through the pilot interventions, an understanding of the benefits of holistic and integrated approaches to support the well-being of older adults, and the need to overcome silos, were reported at all levels, from local communities to care providers and primary care practitioners, up to local and national authorities.

Capacity building and workforce development. Core training modules, adapted to local contexts, equipped care providers, primary care workers, social workers, and community groups and volunteers with knowledge and skills in case management, outreach and home care services, active aging, and common clinical conditions. Benchmarking visits to Singapore and Thailand and cross-country learning increased knowledge sharing, creating a skilled, collaborative workforce.

Experience to inform home and community care policy. These pilots helped generate data and experience to inform policy and program development. In Indonesia, the replication of CCHs by local government in both pilot provinces has been integrated into the country's medium-term development plan. In Mongolia, lessons from the pilot project informed the 2024 amendments to the Elderly Law. In Viet Nam, the provision of home medical treatment and services as piloted has been integrated into the Health Insurance Law.

Key Lessons Learned

The people who need support most are often homebound. As such, they are often not on the radar of service providers. Most of the cases under the case management system, were found through active case finding. Often clients were bedbound and unable to access health care services and social assistance. The case management service was the mechanism to provide holistic support, and the home care services brought assistance to those who needed it most.

The case management service was the mechanism to provide holistic support, and the home care services brought assistance to those who needed it most.

Most LTC happens in homes and communities, delivered by family, friends, and local caregivers. LTC is often equated with nursing homes, but it is a vibrant spectrum of services designed to support individuals with chronic conditions or disabilities. Formal community-based LTC services—such as in-home support and home care—promote dignity, independence, and social integration; support families; and reduce reliance on institutional settings such as hospital and residential care.

Women use home and community care services more. Most case management clients in all three countries were women, reflecting longer lives, often spent in ill health and widowhood, which meant an absence of spousal care. Active aging programs and services were predominantly used by women, perhaps reflecting greater willingness to socialize and stronger social connections, or the suitability and attractiveness of activities, as well as their greater longevity.

Active aging programs are foundational. Active aging—through physical activity, social engagement, nutrition, and regular health checks—empowers older adults to maintain their independence and resilience. Community programs that promote active aging can reduce the onset and severity of chronic conditions, potentially reducing the need for intensive LTC services and fostering vibrant, healthy aging. Many of these programs can be organized simply and at low cost by volunteer and community groups, offered in partnership through CCHs.

LTC needs a blend of professional, family, and community care. Effective LTC needs highly accessible inputs from appropriately trained and coordinated social and health care providers incentivized to work as a team, leveraging the older peoples' strengths while prioritizing their goals when managing noncommunicable diseases (NCDs), and psychosocial and functional impairment. Professionals are required to ensure appropriate care is provided to individuals, especially those with complex conditions.

Structured incentives mean a stronger community care workforce. Community care workers and volunteers play a critical role in delivering community-based LTC, allowing professionals to focus on the most critical and/or complex tasks. The pilots paid honoraria to community care workers to recognize their work and cover out-of-pocket expenses such as transport. While there was broad acceptance of the principle of paying community care workers, there is still a heavy reliance on volunteer roles.

Continuous mentoring and structured support for LTC workforce. Regular training ensures staff stay updated on best practices. Mentoring fosters professional growth, builds confidence, addresses challenges, and reduces burnout and turnover. A structured support system, including scheduled in-service workshops and mentoring, creates consistency and accountability, and cultivates a resilient, skilled workforce. Ultimately, this enhances LTC outcomes and builds trust in community-based LTC programs.

Effective LTC starts with gatekeeping and stratification. These strategies ensure resources are allocated efficiently, prevent over-servicing, and promote early intervention, thus enhancing equity, sustainability, and quality of care.

Systemic LTC solutions call for complex and adaptive thinking. LTC administrators and professionals must integrate interpersonal skills, systems thinking, and adaptive leadership to address aging populations, fragmented systems, and evolving care demands.

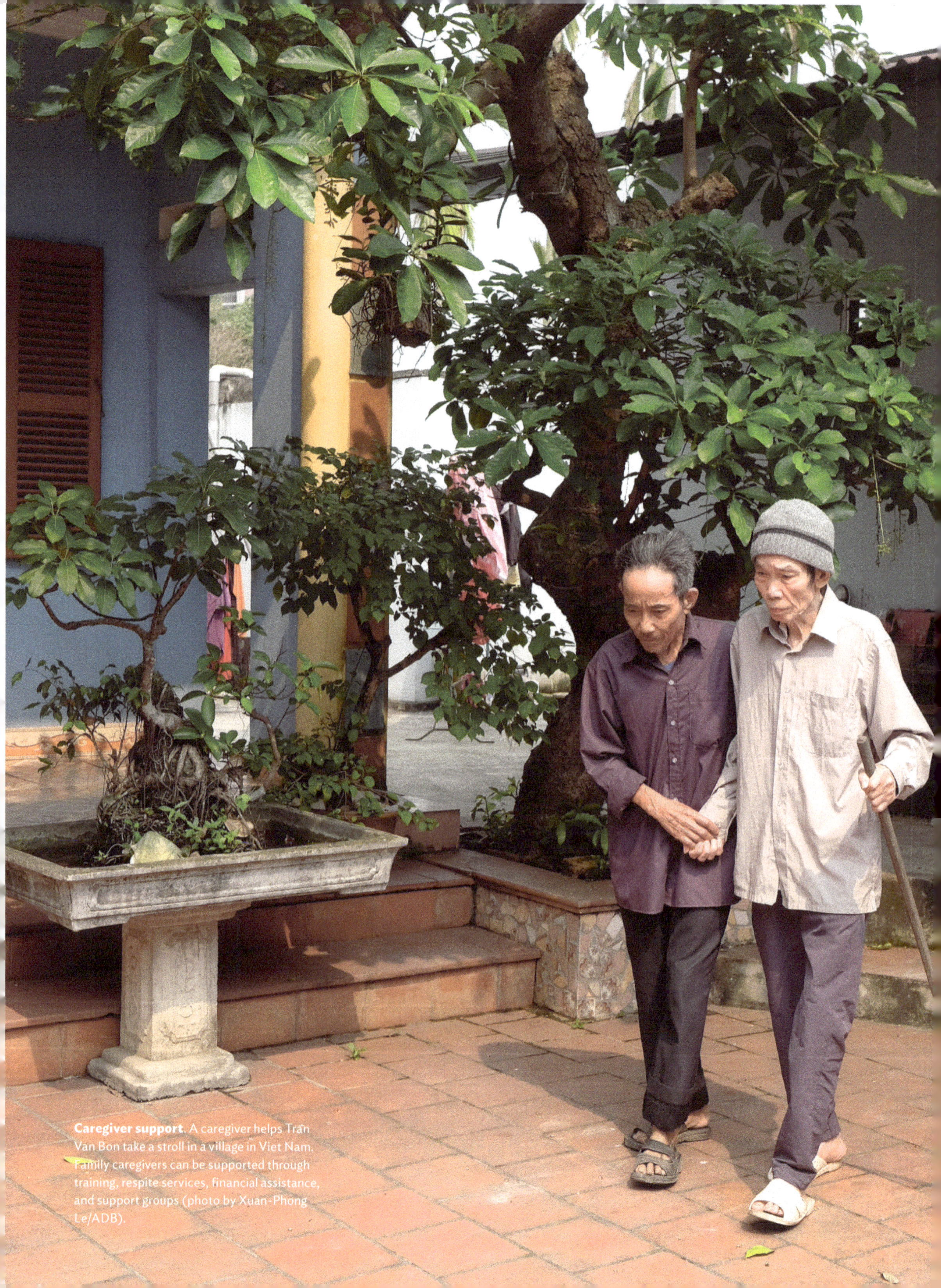

Caregiver support. A caregiver helps Tran Van Bon take a stroll in a village in Viet Nam. Family caregivers can be supported through training, respite services, financial assistance, and support groups (photo by Xuan-Phong Le/ADB).

Strategic Recommendations

Strengthen legal framework for the delivery of community-based LTC. This should include

- clarification of roles across government departments and levels;
- standardization of gatekeeping to access publicly funded LTC services;
- standardization of comprehensive needs assessment with robust data management policies;
- establishment of a quality management framework;
- creation of a work skills qualification framework for professionals, community care workers, and volunteers;
- establishment of local government accountability for the delivery and quality of community-based care; and
- creation of platforms for public and user participation in policy related to community-based care.

Finance community-based LTC. The central government should implement a comprehensive financing strategy, including

- incorporating LTC services into social protection systems, via tax-financed or mandated social insurance schemes or to provide subsidized access for eligible individuals, particularly low- and middle-income populations;
- gatekeeping LTC eligibility to ensure equitable access while maintaining fiscal sustainability;
- allocating specific funds within the national budget for LTC services and distributing the funding to local governments based on regional population needs, demographic profiles, and socioeconomic disparities; and
- promoting and regulating funding diversified mechanisms to include public–private partnership tax incentives and allowing community-led fund-raising initiatives with public sector subsidy.

Provide universal access to community-based LTC systems. This calls for

- expansion of pilot models like CCHs and case management teams with local adaptations;
- mobilization of communities for active case finding and risk screening;
- deployment of outreach teams and mobile units to rural areas;
- coordination with primary care centers; and
- subsidization of services such as home help, home care, and home nursing for low-income older adults.

Close the gap for social and health care in community-based LTC. To do this, it is necessary to

- integrate health and social care by connecting family care, primary care, hospitals, and community organizations;
- create age-friendly health centers with case manager desks;
- support family caregivers with respite care and training; and
- leverage volunteer networks for case finding and social support, and partner with community groups to optimize care delivery.

Involve the housing, built environment, and transport sectors in development of community-based LTC. Age-friendly housing and community environment design will significantly enhance the independence, functionality, mobility, and safety of older people. Involving representatives from these sectors early enough in policy formulation, community pilots, training and awareness, and data sharing is essential. Ensure there are sufficient transport options for older adults to access community-based LTC facilities and for outreach teams to reach homebound clients.

Use technology. This entails

- scaling digital case management platforms like Indonesia's SILANI and Mongolia's mobile app,
- implementing telehealth for remote consultations,
- funding assistive technologies and home modifications to support aging in place, and
- addressing digital literacy barriers through training for older adults and caregivers in low-literacy communities.

Develop a robust data management system. This can then be used to guide policy formulation and evidence-informed practices. There needs to be continual review and enhancement of the digitization of case management systems, such as SILANI in Indonesia, to ensure that data is of sufficient quality to be analyzed to inform policy and practices. Policymakers should collaborate with research institutions to make use of data to support the growth and development of LTC services, as well as the expertise of local researchers.

Build capacity and knowledge for a skilled LTC workforce. Key actions include

- developing accredited case manager training curricula;
- mandating training for professionals and nonprofessionals;
- launching caregiver certification programs, including a focus on dementia and frailty care;
- diversifying LTC teams with specialists like rehabilitation experts; and
- learning for volunteers and knowledge-sharing platforms with research centers.

Promote active aging for healthier communities. This can be through a variety of measures

- promoting active aging through diet, exercise, and stress management workshops;
- supporting recreational and volunteering activities;
- engaging communities in health education;
- implementing preventive care targeting falls and NCDs, and fostering intergenerational activities to reduce social isolation and enhance psychosocial well-being.

Strengthen family caregiver support programs. This calls for action to institutionalize comprehensive family caregiver support, including training, respite services, financial assistance, and support groups. These measures, tailored to local contexts, embed ongoing support for family caregivers in the LTC system. They will enhance caregiver capacity, reduce their burden and burnout, and make LTC more sustainable.

Increase options and accessibility for residential care. Scale-up of integrated and tiered care models could delay institutionalization, reduce pressure on limited residential facilities, and increase accessibility by reserving it for high-need cases. This, in turn, would build a more equitable and efficient home and community care system, while informing strategic investment in residential care infrastructure where necessary.

www.ingramcontent.com/pod-product-compliance
Lightning Source LLC
Chambersburg PA
CBHW041759220926
51847CB00014B/258
* 9 7 8 9 2 9 2 7 7 5 0 3 2 *